Reason To Be Healthy

Contents:

Introduction

Everybody, including health experts agree that there are major benefits of physical activity and proper nutrition. For example, we all agree that regular physical activity reduces the risk of many adverse health outcomes, that some physical activity is better than none, that for most health outcomes, additional benefits occur as the amount of physical activity increases through higher intensity, greater frequency, and/or longer duration. It is also understood that most health benefits occur with at least 2 hours a week of moderately intense physical activity, such as a brisk walk.

We also agree anyone can have more benefits when they increase their physical activity in endurance activities such as aerobics and in muscle-strengthening resistance training. Health and physical benefits are not restricted to any given group of people within our society but for all people, such as children, adolescents, young and middle-aged adults, older adults, as well as for men, women, people with disabilities and all kinds of people across the world. In fact, the benefits we all derive from physical activity and healthy lifestyle far outweigh the possibility of adverse outcomes.

We clearly know enough now to recommend that everybody that value their life should engage in regular physical activity to improve overall health and to reduce risk of many health problems. Physical activity is a leading example of how lifestyle choices have a profound effect on health. The choices we make about other lifestyle factors, such as diet, smoking, and alcohol use, also have important and independent effects on our health.

The primary focus of this little book is to help everybody in setting an easy workable physical and healthy activity that can be carried out every day, every week with minimal effort and enjoyment. The guidelines provided are designed to provide information and guidance on the types and amounts of physical activity that provide substantial health benefits to interested members of the public. The main idea behind the booklet is that regular physical activity over months and years can produce long-term health benefits. Realizing these benefits requires physical activity each week.

A final very important reason behind the guidelines include the fact that most deaths occurring especially within our towns, cities, states, country as well as across the world have been due mainly to risks associated with inactivity.

The good news is that we can all set personal goals for physical activity. Setting these goals involves questions like: "How physically fit do I want to be?" "How important is it to me to reduce my risk of heart disease and diabetes?" "How important is it to me to reduce my risk of falls and hip fracture?" "How much weight do I want to lose and keep off?"

Or "How can physical activity give me a chance to have fun, or be with friends and family?" "Or enjoy the outdoors and improve my personal appearance?" For whatever the reason, the time is NOW!

Guidelines for Physical and Health Benefits for the whole family

Everybody believes we should be regularly physically active to improve overall health and fitness and to prevent many adverse health outcomes. The benefits of physical activity occur in generally healthy people, in people at risk of developing chronic diseases, and in people with current chronic conditions or disabilities. Research tells us about the overwhelming benefits of physical activity and health.

Physical activity affects many health conditions, and the specific amounts and types of activity that benefit each condition vary. Although some health benefits seem to begin with as little as 60 minutes (1 hour) a week, research shows that a total amount of 2 hours and 30 minutes a week of moderate-intensity aerobic activity, such as brisk walking, consistently reduces the risk of many chronic diseases and other adverse health outcomes.

Relationship between Physical Activity and Health

Exercise is a form of physical activity that is planned, structured, repetitive, and performed with the goal of improving health or fitness. So, although all exercise is physical activity, not all physical activity is exercise. Studies have examined the role of physical activity in many groups—men and women, children, teens, adults, older adults, people with disabilities, and women during pregnancy and the postpartum period. These studies have focused on the role that physical activity plays in many health outcomes, including:

- Premature (early) death;

- Diseases such as coronary heart disease, stroke, some cancers, type 2 diabetes, osteoporosis, and depression;

- Risk factors for disease, such as high blood pressure and high blood cholesterol;

- Physical fitness, such as aerobic capacity, and muscle strength and endurance;

- Functional capacity (the ability to engage in activities needed for daily living);

- Mental health, such as depression and cognitive function; and

- Injuries or sudden heart attacks.

Aerobic Activity

In this kind of physical activity (also called an endurance activity or cardio activity), the body's large muscles move in a rhythmic manner for a sustained period of time. Brisk walking, running, bicycling, jumping rope, and swimming are all examples Aerobic activity causes a person's heart to beat faster than usual.

Aerobic physical activity has three components:

•   *Intensity*, or how hard a person works to do the activity. The intensities most often examined are moderate intensity (equivalent in effort to brisk walking) and vigorous intensity (equivalent in effort to running or jogging);

•   *Frequency,* or how often a person does aerobic activity; and

•   *Duration,* or how long a person does an activity in any one session.

Although these components make up a physical activity profile, research has shown that the total amount of physical activity (minutes of moderate intensity physical activity, for example) is more important for achieving health benefits than is any one component (frequency, intensity, or duration).

Muscle-Strengthening Activity

This kind of activity, which includes resistance training and lifting weights, causes the body's muscles to work or hold against an applied force or weight. These activities often involve relatively heavy objects, such as weights, which are lifted multiple times to train various muscle groups. Muscle-strengthening activity can also be done by using elastic bands or body weight for resistance (climbing a tree or doing push-ups, for example).

Muscle-strengthening activity also has three components:

•   *Intensity*, or how much weight or force is used relative to how much a person is able to lift;
•   *Frequency,* or how often a person does muscle strengthening activity; and

•   *Repetitions,* or how many times a person lifts a weight (analogous to duration for aerobic activity).

The effects of muscle-strengthening activity are limited to the muscles doing the work. It's important to work all the major muscle groups of the body: the legs, hips, back, abdomen, chest, shoulders, and arms.

Bone-Strengthening Activity

This kind of activity (sometimes called weight-bearing or weight-loading activity) produces a force on the bones that promotes bone growth and strength. This force is commonly produced by impact with the ground. Examples of bone-strengthening activity include jumping jacks, running, brisk walking, and weight-lifting exercises. As these examples illustrate, bone-strengthening activities can also be aerobic and muscle strengthening.

The Health Benefits of Physical Activity

Studies clearly demonstrate that participating in regular physical activity provides many health benefits. Many conditions affected by physical activity occur with increasing age, such as heart disease and cancer. Reducing risk of these conditions may require years of participation in regular physical activity. However, other benefits, such as increased cardio respiratory fitness, increased muscular strength, and decreased depressive symptoms and blood pressure, require only a few weeks or months of participation in physical activity.

The health benefits of physical activity are seen in children and adolescents, young and middle-aged adults, older adults, women and men, people of different races and ethnicities, and people with disabilities and chronic conditions. The health benefits of physical activity are generally independent of body weight. Adults of all sizes and shapes gain health and fitness benefits by being habitually physically active. The benefits of physical activity also outweigh the risk of injury and sudden heart attacks, two concerns that prevent many people from becoming physically active.

The following sections provide more detail on what is known from research studies about the specific health benefits of physical activity and how much physical activity is needed to get the health benefits.

Premature Death

Strong scientific evidence shows that physical activity reduces the risk of premature death (dying earlier than the average age of death for a specific population group) from the leading causes of death, such as heart disease and some cancers, as well as from other causes of death. This effect is remarkable in two ways:

- First, only a few lifestyle choices have as large an effect on mortality as physical activity. It has been estimated that people who are physically active for approximately 7 hours a week have a 40 percent lower risk of dying early than those who are active for less than 30 minutes a week.

- Second, it is not necessary to do high amounts of activity or vigorous-intensity activity to reduce the risk of premature death. Studies show substantially lower risk when people do 2 and half hours of at least moderate-intensity aerobic physical activity a week

Research clearly demonstrates the importance of avoiding inactivity. Even low amounts of physical activity reduce the risk of dying prematurely. The most dramatic difference in risk is seen between those who are inactive (30 minutes a week) and those with low levels of activity (90 minutes or 1 hour and 30 minutes a week).

The relative risk of dying prematurely continues to be lower with higher levels of reported moderate- or vigorous-intensity leisure-time physical activity. All adults can gain this health benefit of physical activity. Age, race, and ethnicity do not matter. Men and women younger than 65 years as well as older adults have lower rates of early death when they are physically active than when they are inactive.

Physically active people of all body weights (normal weight, overweight, obese) also have lower rates of early death than do inactive people.

Cardio respiratory Health

The benefits of physical activity on cardio respiratory health are some of the most extensively documented of all the health benefits. Cardio respiratory health involves the health of the heart, lungs, and blood vessels.

Heart diseases and stroke are two of the leading causes of death in the United States. Risk factors that increase the likelihood of cardiovascular diseases include smoking, high blood pressure (called hypertension), type 2 diabetes, and high levels of certain blood lipids (such as low-density lipoprotein, or LDL, cholesterol).

Low cardio respiratory fitness also is a risk factor for heart disease. People who do moderate- or vigorous-intensity aerobic physical activity have a significantly lower risk of cardiovascular disease than do inactive people. Regularly active adults have lower rates of heart disease and stroke, and have lower blood pressure, better blood lipid profiles, and fitness. Significant reductions in risk of cardiovascular disease occur at activity levels equivalent to 150 minutes a week of moderate-intensity physical activity. Even greater benefits are seen with 200 minutes (3 hours and 20 minutes) a week. The evidence is strong that greater amounts of physical activity result in even further reductions in the risk of cardiovascular disease.

Everyone can gain the cardiovascular health benefits of physical activity. The amount of physical activity that provides favorable cardio respiratory health and fitness outcomes is similar for adults of various ages, including older people, as well as for adults of various races and ethnicities. Aerobic exercise also improves cardio respiratory fitness in individuals with some disabilities, including people who have lost the use of one or both legs and those with multiple sclerosis, stroke, spinal cord injury, and cognitive disabilities.

Moderate-intensity physical activity is safe for generally healthy women during pregnancy. It increases cardio respiratory fitness without increasing the risk of early pregnancy loss, preterm delivery, or low birth weight. Physical activity during the postpartum period also improves cardio respiratory fitness.

Metabolic Health

Regular physical activity strongly reduces the risk of developing type 2 diabetes as well as the metabolic syndrome. The metabolic syndrome is defined as a condition in which people have some combination of high blood pressure, a large waistline (abdominal obesity), an adverse blood lipid profile (low levels of high-density lipoprotein [HDL] cholesterol, raised triglycerides), and impaired glucose tolerance.

People who regularly engage in at least moderate intensity aerobic activity have a significantly lower risk of developing type 2 diabetes than do inactive people. Although some experts debate the usefulness of defining the metabolic syndrome, good evidence exists that physical activity reduces the risk of having this condition, as defined in various ways. Lower rates of these conditions are seen with 120 to 150 minutes (2 hours to 2 hours and 30 minutes) a week of at least moderate-intensity aerobic activity.

As with cardiovascular health, additional levels of physical activity seem to lower risk even further. In addition, physical activity helps control blood glucose levels in persons who already have type 2 diabetes. Physical activity also improves metabolic health in youth. Studies find this effect when young people participate in at least 3 days of vigorous aerobic activity a week. More physical activity is associated with improved metabolic health, but research has yet to determine the exact amount of improvement. Sclerosis, stroke, spinal cord injury, and cognitive disabilities.

Moderate-intensity physical activity is safe for generally healthy women during pregnancy. It increases cardio respiratory fitness without increasing the risk of early pregnancy loss, preterm delivery, or low birth weight. Physical activity during the postpartum period also improves cardio respiratory fitness.

Obesity and Energy Balance

Overweight and obesity occur when fewer calories are expended, including calories burned through physical activity, than are taken in through food and beverages. Physical activity and caloric intake both must be considered when trying to control body weight. Because of this role in energy balance, physical activity is a critical factor in determining whether a person can maintain a healthy body weight, lose excess body weight, or maintain successful weight loss.

People vary a great deal in how much physical activity they need to achieve and maintain a healthy weight. Some need more physical activity than others to maintain a healthy body weight, to lose weight, or to keep weight off once it has been lost.

Strong scientific evidence shows that physical activity helps people maintain a stable weight over time. However, the optimal amount of physical activity needed to maintain weight is unclear. People vary greatly in how much physical activity results in weight stability. Many people need more than the equivalent of 150 minutes of moderate-intensity activity a week to maintain their weight.

Over short periods of time, such as a year, research shows that it is possible to achieve weight stability by doing the equivalent of 150 to 300 minutes (5 hours) a week of moderate-intensity walking at about a 4 mile-an-hour pace. Muscle-strengthening activities may help promote weight maintenance, although not to the same degree as aerobic activity.

People who want to lose a substantial (more than 5 percent of body weight) amount of weight and people who are trying to keep a significant amount of weight off once it has been lost need a high amount of physical activity unless they also reduce their caloric intake. Many people need to do more than 300 minutes of moderate-intensity activity a week to meet weight control goals.

Regular physical activity also helps control the percentage of body fat in children and adolescents. Exercise training studies with overweight and obese youth have shown that they can reduce their body fatness by participating in physical activity that is at least moderate intensity on 3 to 5 days a week, for 30 to 60 minutes each time.

Musculoskeletal Health

Bones, muscles, and joints support the body and help it move. Healthy bones, joints, and muscles are critical to the ability to do daily activities without physical limitations.

Preserving bone, joint, and muscle health is essential with increasing age. Studies show that the frequent decline in bone density that happens during aging can be slowed with regular physical activity. These effects are seen in people who participate in aerobic, muscle strengthening, and bone-strengthening physical activity programs of moderate or vigorous intensity. The range of total physical activity for these benefits varies widely. Important changes seem to begin at 90 minutes a week and continue up to 5 hours a week.

Hip fracture is a serious health condition that can have life-changing negative effects for many older people. Physically active people, especially women, appear to have a lower risk of hip fracture than do inactive people. Research studies on physical activity to prevent hip fracture show that participating in 120 to 5 hours a week of physical activity that is of at least moderate intensity is associated with a reduced risk. It is unclear, however, whether activity also lowers risk of fractures of the spine or other important areas of the skeleton.

Building strong, healthy bones is also important for children and adolescents. Along with having a healthy diet that includes adequate calcium and vitamin D, physical activity is critical for bone development in children and adolescents. Bone-strengthening physical activity done 3 or more days a week increases bone mineral content and bone density in youth.

Regular physical activity also helps people with arthritis or other rheumatic conditions affecting the joints. Participation in 130 to 150 minutes (2 hours and 10 minutes to 2 hours and 30 minutes) a week of moderate-intensity, low-impact physical activity improves pain management, function, and quality of life. Researchers don't yet know whether participation in physical activity, particularly at low to moderate intensity, reduces the risk of osteoarthritis. Very high levels of physical activity, however, may have extra risks. People who participate in very high levels of physical activity, such as elite or professional athletes, have a higher risk of hip and knee osteoarthritis, mostly due to the risk of injury involved in competing in some sports.

Progressive muscle-strengthening activities increase or preserve muscle mass, strength, and power. Higher amounts (through greater frequency or higher weights) improve muscle function to a greater degree. Improvements occur in younger and older adults. Resistance exercises also improve muscular strength in persons with such conditions as stroke, multiple sclerosis, cerebral palsy, spinal cord injury, and cognitive disability. Though it doesn't increase muscle mass in the same way that muscle-strengthening activities do, aerobic activity may also help slow the loss of muscle with aging.

Functional Ability and Fall Prevention

Functional ability is the capacity of a person to perform tasks or behaviors that enable him or her to carry out everyday activities, such as climbing stairs or walking on a sidewalk. Functional ability is key to a person's ability to fulfill basic life roles, such as personal care, grocery shopping, or playing with the grandchildren. Loss of functional ability is referred to as functional limitation.

Middle-aged and older adults who are physically active have lower risk of functional limitations than do inactive adults. It appears that greater physical activity levels can further reduce risk of functional limitations. Older adults who already have functional limitations also benefit from regular physical activity.

Typically, studies of physical activity in adults with functional limitations tested a combination of aerobic and muscle strengthening activities, making it difficult to assess the relative importance of each type of activity. However, both types of activity appear to provide benefit.

In older adults at risk of falls, strong evidence shows that regular physical activity is safe and reduces this risk. Reduction in falls is seen for participants in programs that include balance and moderate-intensity muscle-strengthening activities for 90 minutes a week plus moderate-intensity walking for about an hour a week. It's not known whether different combinations of type, amount, or frequency of activity can reduce falls to a greater degree. Tai chi exercises also may help prevent falls.

Cancer

Physically active people have a significantly lower risk of colon cancer than do inactive people, and physically active women have a significantly lower risk of breast cancer. Research shows that a wide range of moderate-intensity physical activity—between 210 and 420 minutes a week (3 hours and 30 minutes to 7 hours)—is needed to significantly reduce the risk of colon and breast cancer; currently, 150 minutes a week does not appear to provide a major benefit. It also appears that greater amounts of physical activity lower risks of these cancers even further, although exactly how much lower is not clear.

Although not definitive, some research suggests that the risk of endometrial cancer in women and lung cancers in men and women also may be lower among those who are regularly active compared to those who are inactive.

Finally, cancer survivors have a better quality of life and improved physical fitness if they are physically active, compared to survivors who are inactive.

Mental Health

Physically active adults have lower risk of depression and cognitive decline (declines with aging in thinking, learning, and judgment skills). Physical activity also may improve the quality of sleep. Whether physical activity reduces distress or anxiety is currently unclear. Mental health benefits have been found in people who do aerobic or a combination of aerobic and muscle strengthening activities 3 to 5 days a week for 30 to 60 minutes at a time. Some research has shown that even lower levels of physical activity also may provide some benefits.

Regular physical activity appears to reduce symptoms of anxiety and depression for children and adolescents. Whether physical activity improves self-esteem is not clear.

Adverse Events

Some people hesitate to become active or increase their level of physical activity because they fear getting injured or having a heart attack. Studies of generally healthy people clearly show that moderate-intensity physical activity, such as brisk walking, has a low risk of such adverse events. The risk of musculoskeletal injury increases with the total amount of physical activity. For example, a person who regularly runs 40 miles a week has a higher risk of injury than a person who runs 10 miles each week. However, people who are physically active may

have fewer injuries from other causes, such as motor vehicle collisions or work-related injuries. Depending on the type and amount of activity that physically active people do, their overall injury rate may be lower than the overall injury rate for inactive people.

Participation in contact or collision sports, such as soccer or football, has a higher risk of injury than participation in non-contact physical activity, such as swimming or walking. However, when performing the same activity, people who are less it are more likely to be injured than people who are fitter.

Cardiac events, such as a heart attack or sudden death during physical activity, are rare. However, the risk of such cardiac events does increase when a person suddenly becomes much more active than usual.

The greatest risk occurs when an adult who is usually inactive engages in vigorous-intensity activity (such as shoveling snow). People who are regularly physically active have the lowest risk of cardiac events both while being active and overall.

The bottom line is that the health benefits of physical activity far outweigh the risks of adverse events for almost everyone.

Health Benefits Associated With Regular Physical Activity

Children and Adolescents Strong evidence

- Improved cardio respiratory and muscular fitness
- Improved bone health
- Improved cardiovascular and metabolic health biomarkers
- Favorable body composition

Moderate evidence

- Reduced symptoms of depression

Adults and Older Adults
Strong evidence

- Lower risk of early death

- Lower risk of coronary heart disease

- Lower risk of stroke

- Lower risk of high blood pressure

- Lower risk of adverse blood lipid profile

- Lower risk of type 2 diabetes

- Lower risk of metabolic syndrome

- Lower risk of colon cancer

- Lower risk of breast cancer

- Prevention of weight gain

- Weight loss, particularly when combined with reduced

calorie intake

- Improved cardio respiratory and muscular fitness

- Prevention of falls

- Reduced depression

- Better cognitive function (for older adults)

Moderate to strong evidence

- Better functional health (for older adults)

- Reduced abdominal obesity

Moderate evidence

- Lower risk of hip fracture

- Lower risk of lung cancer

- Lower risk of endometrial cancer

- Weight maintenance after weight loss

- Increased bone density

- Improved sleep quality

The Beneficial Effects of Increasing Physical Activity: It's About Overload, Progression, and Specificity

Overload is the physical stress placed on the body when physical activity is greater in amount or intensity than usual. The body's structures and functions respond and adapt to these stresses. For example, aerobic physical activity places a stress on the cardio respiratory system and muscles, requiring the lungs to move more air and the heart to pump more blood and deliver it to the working muscles. This increase in demand increases the efficiency and capacity of the lungs, heart, circulatory system, and exercising muscles. In the same way, muscle strengthening and bone-strengthening activities overload muscles and bones, making them stronger.

Progression is closely tied to overload. Once a person reaches a certain fitness level, he or she progresses to higher levels of physical activity by continued overload and adaptation. Small, progressive changes in overload help the body adapt to the additional stresses while minimizing the risk of injury.

Specificity means that the benefits of physical activity are specific to the body systems that are doing the work. For example, aerobic physical activity largely benefits the body's cardiovascular system.

Guidelines for Children and Adolescents

In general children and adolescents can benefit from an hour or more daily physical activity such as aerobics, which could be either moderate or vigorous to intense and could include vigorous to intense physical activity for up to three days a week. As part of the one hour daily physical activity, children and adolescents can include muscle strengthening physical activity during the three day weekly exercise. Bone strength building physical activity should be included in the routine mentioned above on a daily and weekly basis.

As parents, family, and educators, we can build a great long term habit through support and encouragement of young people to participate in physical activities that are appropriate
for their age, that are enjoyable, and that offer variety.

Regular physical activity in children and adolescents promotes health and fitness. Compared to those who are inactive, physically active youth have higher levels of cardio respiratory fitness and stronger muscles. They also typically have lower body fatness. Their bones are stronger, and they may have reduced symptoms of anxiety and depression.

According to health experts, youth who are regularly active also have a better chance of a healthy adulthood. Children and adolescents don't usually develop chronic diseases, such as heart disease, hypertension, type 2 diabetes, or osteoporosis. However, risk factors for these diseases can begin to develop early in life. Regular physical activity makes it less likely that these risk factors will develop and more likely that children will remain healthy as adults.

Children and Adolescents can achieve substantial health benefits by doing moderate- and vigorous-intensity physical activity for periods of time that add up to 1 hour or more each day. This activity should include aerobic activity as well as age-appropriate muscle- and bones strengthening activities. Bone-strengthening activities remain especially important for children and young adolescents because the greatest gains in bone mass occur during the years just before and during puberty.

Since the majority of peak bone mass is obtained by the end of adolescence, adults and parents who work with or take care of youth should know that they play an important role in providing
age-appropriate opportunities for physical activity. In doing so, they help lay an important foundation for life-long, health-promoting physical activity. Adults need to encourage active play in children and encourage sustained and structured activity as children grow older.

Types of Activity

Three major activities for children and adolescents should focus on: aerobic, muscle-strengthening, and bone-strengthening. Each type has important health benefits.
•   Aerobic activities are those in which young people rhythmically move their large muscles. Running, hopping, skipping, jumping rope, swimming, dancing, and bicycling are all examples of aerobic activities. Aerobic activities increase cardio respiratory fitness. Children often do activities in short bursts, which may not technically be aerobic activities. However, this document will also use the term aerobic to refer to these brief activities.
•   Muscle-strengthening activities make muscles do more work than .usual during activities
of daily life. This is called "overload," and it strengthens the muscles. Muscle-strengthening activities can be unstructured and part of play, such as playing on playground equipment, climbing trees, and playing tug-of-war. Or these activities can be structured, such as lifting weights or working with resistance band.
•   Bone-strengthening activities produce a force on the bones that promotes bone growth and strength. This force is commonly produced by impact with the ground. Running, jumping rope, basketball, tennis, and hopscotch are all examples of bone strengthening activities. Its important to know that bone-strengthening activities can also be aerobic and muscle-strengthening.

Physical Activity and Healthy Weight

Regular physical activity in children and adolescents promotes a healthy body weight and body composition. Exercise training in overweight or obese youth can improve body composition by reducing overall levels of fatness as well as abdominal fatness. Research studies report that fatness can be reduced by regular physical activity of moderate to vigorous intensity 3 to 5 times a week, for 30 to 60 minutes.

Meeting Guidelines

To meet the Guidelines, we have to understand that children and adolescents vary in their physical activity participation. Some don't participate at all. Others participate in enough activity to meet the Guidelines, and some exceed the Guidelines.

One practical strategy to promote activity in youth is to replace inactivity with activity whenever possible. For example, where appropriate and safe, young people should walk or bicycle to school instead of riding in a car. Rather than just watching sporting events on television, young people should participate in age appropriate sports or games.
•   Children and adolescents who do not meet the Guidelines should slowly increase their activity in small steps and in ways that they enjoy. A gradual increase in the number of days and the time spent being active will help reduce the risk of injury.
•   Children and adolescents who meet the Guidelines should continue being active on a daily basis and, if appropriate, become even more active. Evidence suggests that even more than 60 minutes of activity every day may provide additional health benefits.
•   Children and adolescents who exceed the Guidelines should maintain their activity level and vary the kinds of activities they do to reduce the risk of overtraining or injury.

Children and adolescents with disabilities are more likely to be inactive than those without disabilities. Youth with disabilities should work with their healthcare provider to understand the types and amounts of physical activity appropriate for them. When possible, children and adolescents with disabilities should meet the Guidelines. When young people are not able to participate in appropriate physical activities to meet the Guidelines, they should be as active as possible and avoid being inactive.

Key Guidelines for Children and Adolescents

•   Children and adolescents should do 60 minutes (1 hour) or more of physical activity daily.

—   Aerobic: Most of the 60 or more minutes a day should be either moderate- or vigorous-intensity aerobic physical activity, and should include vigorous-intensity physical activity at least 3 days a week.

— Muscle-strengthening: As part of their 60 or more minutes of daily physical activity, children and adolescents should include muscle-strengthening physical activity on at least 3 days of the week.

— Bone-strengthening: As part of their 60 or more minutes of daily physical activity, children and adolescents should include bone-strengthening physical activity on at least 3 days of the week.

• It is important to encourage young people to participate in physical activities that are appropriate for their age, that are enjoyable, and that offer variety

Examples

Children and adolescents can meet the Physical Activity Guidelines and become regularly physically active in many ways. Here are just two examples showing how a child and an adolescent can be physically active for at least 60 minutes each day over the course of a week.

These examples illustrate that even though the activity patterns are different, each young person is meeting the Guidelines by getting the equivalent of at least 60 minutes or more of aerobic activity each day that is at least moderate intensity. Both are also doing vigorous-intensity, muscle-strengthening, and bone strengthening activities on at least 3 days a week.

- **Harold: A 7-Year-Old Child**

Harold participates in many types of physical activities in many places. For example, during physical education class, he jumps rope and does gymnastics and sit-ups.
During recess, he plays on the playground—often by doing activities that require running and climbing. He also likes to play soccer with his friends and family. When Harold gets home from school, he likes to engage in active play (playing tag) and ride his bicycle with his friends and family. Harold gets 60 minutes of physical activity each day that is at least moderate intensity. He participates in the following activities each day:

Monday: Walks to and from school (20 minutes), plays actively with family (20 minutes), jumps rope (10 minutes), does gymnastics (10 minutes).

Tuesday: Walks to and from school (20 minutes), plays on playground (25 minutes), climbs on playground equipment (15 minutes).

Wednesday: Walks to and from school (20 minutes), plays actively with friends (25 minutes), jumps rope (10 minutes), runs (5 minutes), does sit-ups (2 minutes).

Thursday: Plays actively with family (30 minutes), plays soccer (30 minutes).

Friday: Walks to and from school (20 minutes), plays actively with friends (25 minutes), bicycles (15 minutes).

Saturday: Plays on playground (30 minutes), climbs on playground equipment (15 minutes), bicycles (15 minutes).

Sunday: Plays on playground (10 minutes), plays soccer (40 minutes), plays tag with family (10 minutes).

Harold meets the Guidelines by doing vigorous intensity aerobic activities, bone-strengthening activities, and muscle-strengthening activities on at least 3 days of the week:

• Vigorous-intensity aerobic activities 6 times during the week: jumping rope (Monday and Wednesday), running (Wednesday), soccer (Thursday and Sunday), playing tag (Sunday);

• Bone-strengthening activities 6 times during the week: jumping rope (Monday and Wednesday), running (Wednesday), soccer (Thursday and Sunday), playing tag (Sunday); and

• Muscle-strengthening activities 4 times during the week: gymnastics (Monday), climbing on playground equipment (Tuesday and Saturday), sit-ups (Wednesday).

- **Maria: A 16-Year-Old Adolescent**

Maria participates in many types of physical activities in many places. For example, during physical education class, she plays tennis and does sit-ups and push-ups. She also likes to play basketball at the YMCA, do yoga, and go dancing with friends. Maria likes to take her dog on walks and hikes. Maria gets 60 or more minutes of daily physical activity that is at least moderate intensity. She participates in the following activities each day:

Monday: Walks dog (10 minutes), plays basketball at YMCA (50 minutes).

Tuesday: Walks dog (10 minutes), plays tennis (30 minutes), does sit-ups and push-ups (5 minutes), walks briskly with friends (15 minutes).

Wednesday: Walks dog (10 minutes), plays basketball at YMCA (50 minutes).

Thursday: Walks dog (10 minutes), plays tennis (30 minutes), does sit-ups and push-ups (5 minutes), plays with children at the park while babysitting (15 minutes).

Friday: Plays Frisbee® in park (45 minutes), mows lawn (30 minutes).

Saturday: Goes dancing with friends (60 minutes), does yoga (30 minutes).

Sunday: Hikes (60 minutes).

Maria meets the Guidelines by doing vigorous-intensity aerobic activities, bone-strengthening activities, and muscle-strengthening activities on at least 3 days of the week:

•   Vigorous-intensity aerobic activities 4 times during the week: basketball (Monday and Wednesday), dancing (Saturday), hiking (Sunday);

•   Bone-strengthening activities 4 times during the week: basketball (Monday and Wednesday), dancing (Saturday), hiking (Sunday); and

•   Muscle-strengthening activities 3 times during the week: sit-ups and push-ups (Tuesday and Thursday), yoga (Saturday*)*.

Guidelines for Adults

For adults to maximize the benefits of physical and healthy activities, they should avoid inactivity. Some physical activity is better than none, and adults who participate in any amount of physical activity gain some health benefits. For substantial health benefits, adults should do at least a little over 2 hours a week of moderate-intensity, a week of vigorous-intensity aerobic physical activity, or an equivalent combination of moderate- and vigorous-intensity aerobic activity. Aerobic activity can be performed in episodes of at least 10 minutes, and preferably, it can be spread throughout the week. For additional and more extensive health benefits, adults can increase their aerobic physical activity to approximately half dozen hours a week of moderate intensity, or a little over 2 hours a week of vigorous intensity aerobic physical activity, or an equivalent combination of moderate- and vigorous-intensity activity. Of course, more health benefits are gained by engaging in physical activity beyond this amount. Additionally, adults can engage in muscle-strengthening activities that are moderate or high intensity and involve all major muscle groups on 2 or more days a week, as these activities provide additional health benefits.

Adults who are physically active are healthier and less likely to develop many chronic diseases than adults who are inactive. They also have better fitness, including a healthier body size and composition. These benefits are gained by men and women and people of all races, ethnicities, and nationalities.

Adults gain most of these health benefits when they do the equivalent of at least over 2 hours of moderate intensity aerobic physical activity (2 hours and 30 minutes) each week. Adults gain additional and more extensive health and fitness benefits with even more physical activity. Muscle-strengthening activities also provide health benefits and are an important part of an adult's overall physical activity plan.

The adult category includes but not limited to most men and women aged 18 to 64 years, and focuses on physical activity beyond baseline activity (the usual light or sedentary activities of daily living). Physical activity guidelines for women during pregnancy and the postpartum period and for adults with disabilities and select chronic conditions are discussed elsewhere.

Types of Activities

The Guidelines for adults focus on two types of activity: *aerobic and muscle-strengthening*. Each type provides important health benefits.

Aerobic Activity
Aerobic activities, also called endurance activities, are physical activities in which people move their large muscles in a rhythmic manner for a sustained period. Running, brisk walking, bicycling, playing basketball, dancing, and swimming are all examples of

aerobic activities. Aerobic activity makes a person's heart beat more rapidly to meet the demands of the body's movement. Over time, regular aerobic activity makes the heart and cardiovascular system stronger and fitter.

The purpose of the aerobic activity does not affect whether it counts toward meeting the Guidelines. For example, physically active occupations can count toward meeting the Guidelines, as can active transportation choices (walking or bicycling). All types of aerobic activities can count as long as they are of sufficient intensity and duration. Time spent in muscle strengthening activities does not count toward the aerobic activity guidelines.

When putting the Guidelines into action, it's important to consider the total amount of activity, as well as how often to be active, for how long, and at what intensity

How Much Total Activity a Week?

When adults do the equivalent of over 2 hours of moderate-intensity aerobic activity each week, the benefits are substantial. These benefits include lower risk of premature death, coronary heart disease, stroke, hypertension, type 2 diabetes, and depression.

Not all health benefits of physical activity occur at over 2 hours a week. As a person moves from over 2 and half hours a week toward 5 hours a week, he or she gains additional health benefits.

Additional benefits include lower risk of colon and breast cancer and prevention of unhealthy weight gain.

Also, as a person moves from 2 and half hours a week toward 5 hours a week, the benefits that occur at 2 and half hours a week become more extensive. For example, a person who does 5 hours a week has an even lower risk of heart disease or diabetes than a person who does 2 and half hours a week.

The benefits continue to increase when a person does more than the equivalent of 5 hours a week of moderate-intensity aerobic activity. For example, a person who does 7 hours a week has an even lower risk of premature death than a person who does 2 and half hours to 5 hours a week.

How Many Days a Week and for How Long?

Aerobic physical activity should preferably be spread throughout the week. Research studies consistently show that activity performed on at least 3 days a week produces health benefits. Spreading physical activity across at least 3 days a week may help to reduce the risk of injury and avoid excessive fatigue.

Both moderate- and vigorous-intensity aerobic activity can be performed in episodes of at least 10 minutes. Episodes of this duration are known to improve cardiovascular fitness and some risk factors for heart disease and type 2 diabetes.

How Intense?

The Guidelines for adults focus on two levels of intensity: moderate-intensity activity and vigorous intensity activity. To meet the Guidelines, adults can do either moderate-intensity or vigorous-intensity aerobic activities, or a combination of both. It takes less time to get the same benefit from vigorous-intensity activities as from moderate-intensity activities. A general rule of thumb is that 2 minutes of moderate-intensity activity counts the same as 1 minute of vigorous-intensity activity. For example, 30 minutes of moderate-intensity activity a week is roughly the same as 15 minutes of vigorous-intensity activity.

Examples of Different Aerobic Physical Activities and Intensities

Moderate Intensity
- Walking briskly (3 miles per hour or faster, but not race-walking)
- Water aerobics
- Bicycling slower than 10 miles per hour
- Tennis (doubles)
- Ballroom dancing
- General gardening

Vigorous Intensity
- Race walking, jogging, or running
- Swimming laps
- Tennis (singles)
- Aerobic dancing
- Bicycling 10 miles per hour or faster
- Jumping rope
- Heavy gardening (continuous digging or hoeing, with heart rate increases)
- Hiking uphill or with a heavy backpacking

Muscle-Strengthening Activity

Muscle-strengthening activities provide additional benefits not found with aerobic activity. The benefits of muscle-strengthening activity include increased bone strength and muscular fitness. Muscle-strengthening activities can also help maintain muscle mass during a program of weight loss. Muscle-strengthening activities make muscles do more work than they are accustomed to doing. That is, they overload the muscles. Resistance training, including weight training, is a familiar example of muscle-strengthening activity.

Other examples include working with resistance bands, doing calisthenics that use body weight for resistance (such as push-ups, pull-ups, and sit-ups), carrying heavy loads, and heavy gardening (such as digging or hoeing).

Muscle-strengthening activities count if they involve a moderate to high level of intensity or effort and work the major muscle groups of the body: the legs, hips, back, chest, abdomen, shoulders, and arms. Muscle strengthening activities for all the major muscle groups should be done at least 2 days a week.

No specific amount of time is recommended for muscle strengthening, but muscle-strengthening exercises should be performed to the point at which it would be difficult to do another repetition without help. When resistance training is used to enhance muscle strength, one set of 8 to 12 repetitions of each exercise is effective, although two or three sets may be more effective. Development of muscle strength and endurance is progressive over time. Increases in the amount of weight or the days a week of exercising will result in stronger muscles

Meeting Guidelines

Adults have many options for becoming physically active, increasing their physical activity, and staying active throughout their lives. In deciding how to meet the Guidelines, adults should think about how much physical activity they're already doing and how physically it they are. Personal health and fitness goals are also important to consider.

In general, healthy men and women who plan prudent increases in their weekly amounts of physical activity do not need to consult a health-care provider before becoming active.
Inactive Adults Inactive adults or those who don't yet do 2 and half hours of physical activity a week should work gradually toward this goal. The initial amount of activity should

be at a light or moderate intensity, for short periods of time, with the sessions spread throughout the week. The good news is that "some is better than none."

People gain some health benefits even when they do as little as 60 minutes a week of moderate-intensity aerobic physical activity.

To reduce risk of injury, it is important to increase the amount of physical activity gradually over a period of weeks to months. For example, an inactive person could start with a walking program consisting of 5 minutes of slow walking several times each day, 5 to 6 days a week.
The length of time could then gradually be increased to 10 minutes per session, 3 times a day, and the walking speed could be increased slowly. Muscle-strengthening activities should also be gradually increased over time. Initially, these activities can be done just 1 day a week starting at a light or moderate level of effort. Over time, the number of days a week can be increased to 2, and then possibly to more than 2. Each week, the level of effort (intensity) can be increased slightly until it becomes moderate to high.

Active Adults

Adults who are already active and meet the minimum Guidelines (the equivalent of 2 and half hours of moderate-intensity aerobic activity every week) can gain additional and more extensive health and fitness benefits by increasing physical activity above this amount. Most adults should increase their aerobic activity to exceed the minimum level and move toward 5 hours a week. Adults should also do muscle-strengthening activities on at least 2 days each week.

One time-efficient way to achieve greater fitness and health goals is to substitute vigorous-intensity aerobic activity for some moderate-intensity activity. Using the 2-to-1 rule of thumb, doing 2 and half hours of vigorous-intensity aerobic activity a week provides about the same benefits as 5 hours of moderate intensity activity. Adults are encouraged to do a variety of activities, as variety probably reduces risk of injury caused by doing too much of one kind of activity (this is called an overuse injury).

Highly Active Adults

Adults who are highly active should maintain their activity level. These adults are also encouraged to do variety of activities.

- Flexibility Activities

Flexibility is an important part of physical fitness. Some types of physical activity, such as dancing, require more flexibility than others. Stretching exercises are effective in increasing flexibility, and thereby can allow people to more easily do activities that require greater flexibility.

For this reason, flexibility activities are an appropriate part of a physical activity program, even though they have no known health benefits and it is unclear whether they reduce risk of injury. Time spent doing flexibility activities by themselves does not count toward meeting the aerobic or muscle-strengthening Guidelines.

Warm-up and Cool-down

Warm-up and cool-down activities are an acceptable part of a person's physical activity plan. Commonly, the warm-up and cool-down involve doing an activity at a slower speed or lower intensity. A warm-up before moderate- or vigorous-intensity aerobic activity allows a gradual increase in heart rate and breathing at the start of the episode of activity. A cool down after activity allows a gradual decrease at the end of the episode. Time spent doing warm-up and cool-down may count toward meeting the aerobic activity Guidelines if the activity is at least moderate intensity (for example, walking briskly as a warm-up before jogging). A warm-up for muscle-strengthening activity commonly involves doing exercises with lighter weight.

Physical Activity in a Weight-Control Plan

Along with appropriate dietary intake, physical activity is an important part of maintaining healthy weight, losing weight, and keeping extra weight off once it has been lost. Physical activity also helps reduce abdominal fat and preserve muscle during weight loss. Adults should aim for a healthy, stable body weight. The amount of physical activity necessary to achieve this weight varies greatly from person to person.

The first step in achieving or maintaining a healthy weight is to meet the minimum level of physical activity in the Guidelines. For some people this will result in a stable and healthy body weight, but for many it may not.

The health benefits of physical activity are generally independent of body weight. The good news for people needing to lose weight is that regular physical activity provides major health benefits, no matter how their weight changes over time.

Adults should strongly consider walking as one good way to get aerobic physical activity. Many studies show that walking has health benefits and a low risk of injury. It can be done year-round and in many settings. People who are at a healthy body weight but slowly gaining weight can either gradually increase the level of physical activity (toward the equivalent of 5 hours a week of moderate-intensity aerobic activity), or reduce caloric intake, or both, until their weight is stable.

By regularly checking body weight, people can find the amount of physical activity that works for them. Many adults will need to do more than the 2 and half hours a week of moderate-intensity aerobic physical activity as part of a program to lose weight or keep it off.

These adults should do more physical activity and/or further reduce their caloric intake. Some people will need to do the equivalent of 5 hours or more minutes of moderate-intensity physical activity a week to meet their weight-control goals. Combined with restricting caloric intake, these adults should gradually increase minutes or the intensity of aerobic physical activity per week, to the point at which the physical activity is effective in achieving a healthy weight.

It is important to remember that all activities—both baseline and physical activity—"count" for energy balance. Active choices, such as taking the stairs rather than the elevator or adding short episodes of walking to the day, are examples of activities that can be helpful in weight control.
For weight control, vigorous-intensity activity is far more time-efficient than moderate-intensity activity.

Examples

For example, an adult who weighs 165 pounds (75 kg) will burn 560 calories from 2 and half hours of brisk walking at 4 miles an hour (these calories are in addition to the calories normally burned by a body at rest). That person can burn the same number of additional calories in 50 minutes by running 5 miles at a 10 minutes-per-mile pace.

Adults can meet the Physical Activity Guidelines in all sorts of ways and with many types of physical activity. The choices of types and amounts of physical activity depend on personal health and fitness goals. Here are three examples.

- **Jean: An Inactive Middle-Aged Woman**

Her goals: Jean sets a goal of doing 1 hour a day of moderate-intensity aerobic activity on 5 days a week (a total of 300 minutes a week). Weighing 220 pounds, Jean is obese and wants to lose about 1 pound of weight each week.

Starting out: Jean cuts back on her caloric intake and starts walking 5 minutes in the morning and 5 minutes in the evening most days of the week. She walks at a 2.5 mile-an-hour pace. Although physical activity tables show this to be light-intensity activity, for her level of fitness and fatness, it is appropriate moderate intensity activity.

Making good progress: Two months later, Jean is comfortably walking 30 to 40 minutes at moderate intensity, to and from her bus stop, every day. She then adds variety to her activity by alternating among walking, riding a stationary cycle, and low-impact aerobics. She also begins muscle-strengthening activities, using elastic bands twice each week.

Reaching her goal: Eventually, Jean works up to 5 hours a week of moderate-intensity aerobic activity, including her brisk walks to and from the bus stop. She has lost 40 pounds of weight in 1 year, with most of the weight loss occurring the previous 6 months when she mastered her diet and was able to do greater amounts of physical activity.

- **Douglas: An Active Middle-Aged Man**

His goal and current activity pattern: Douglas was a soccer player in his youth. His goal is to get back into shape by becoming a regular recreational runner. In addition to his job operating heavy equipment, he walks 30 to 40 minutes a day on 5 days each week. He also lifts weights 2 days a week.

Starting out: Douglas starts a walk/jog program with a co-worker and plans to gradually replace walking with jogging and then running. The first week he goes out on 5 days, walking for 25 minutes and jogging for 5 minutes.

Making good progress: Each week, Douglas gradually increases the time spent jogging (vigorous-intensity activity) and reduces the time spent walking (moderate intensity activity). He also continues his weight-lifting program.

Reaching his goal: Eventually, Douglas is running 30 to 45 minutes 4 days a week and lifting weights 2 days a week. He goes for a 1-hour bicycle ride on most weekends.

- **Anita: A Very Active College-Aged Adult**

Her goals and current activity pattern: Anita plays league basketball (vigorous-intensity activity) 4 days each week for 90 minutes each day. She wants to reduce her risk of injury from doing too much of one kind of activity (this is called an overuse injury).

Starting out: Anita starts out by cutting back her basketball playing to 3 days each week. She begins to bicycle to and from campus (30 minutes each way) instead of driving her car. She also joins a yoga class that meets twice each week.

Reaching her goal: Eventually, Anita is bicycling 3 days each week to and from campus in addition to playing basketball. Her yoga class helps her to build and maintain strength and flexibility.

Achieving Target Levels of Physical Activity: The Possibilities Are Endless

These examples show how it's possible to meet the Guidelines by doing moderate-intensity or vigorous-intensity activity or a combination of both. Physical activity at this level provides substantial health benefits.

Ways to get the equivalent of 2 hours and 30 minutes of moderate-intensity aerobic physical activity a week plus muscle-strengthening activities:

•   Thirty minutes of brisk walking (moderate intensity) on 5 days, exercising with resistance bands (muscle strengthening) on 2 days;

•   Twenty-five minutes of running (vigorous intensity) on 3 days, lifting weights on 2 days (muscle strengthening);

•   Thirty minutes of brisk walking on 2 days, 60 minutes (1 hour) of social dancing (moderate intensity) on 1 evening, 30 minutes of mowing the lawn (moderate intensity) on 1 afternoon, heavy gardening (muscle strengthening) on 2 days;

•   Thirty minutes of an aerobic dance class on 1 morning (vigorous intensity), 30 minutes of running on 1 day (vigorous intensity), 30 minutes of brisk walking on 1 day (moderate intensity), calisthenics (such as sit-ups, push-ups) on 3 days (muscle strengthening);

•   Thirty minutes of biking to and from work on 3 days (moderate intensity), playing softball for 60 minutes on 1 day (moderate intensity), using weight machines on 2 days (muscle-strengthening on 2 days); and
•   Forty-five minutes of doubles tennis on 2 days (moderate intensity), lifting weights after work on 1 day (muscle strengthening), hiking vigorously for 30 minutes and rock climbing (muscle strengthening) on 1 day.

Ways to be even more active

For adults who are already doing at least 150 minutes of moderate-intensity physical activity, here are a few ways to do even more. Physical activity at this level has even greater health benefits:

•   Forty-five minutes of brisk walking every day, exercising with resistance bands on 2 or 3 days;

•   Forty-five minutes of running on 3 or 4 days, circuit weight training in a gym on 2 or 3 days;

- Thirty minutes of running on 2 days, 45 minutes of brisk walking on 1 day, 45 minutes of an aerobics and weights class on 1 day, 90 minutes (1 hour and 30 minutes) of social dancing on 1 evening, 30 minutes of mowing the lawn, plus some heavy garden work on 1 day;

- Ninety minutes of playing soccer on 1 day, brisk walking for 15 minutes on 3 days, lifting weights on 2 days; and

- Forty-five minutes of stationary bicycling on 2 days, 60 minutes of basketball on 2 days, calisthenics on 3 days.

Guidelines for Older Adults

The guidelines for older adults are similar to those of adults. However, the following guidelines are appropriate for older adults: When older adults cannot do over 2 hours of moderate-intensity aerobic activity a week because of chronic conditions, they can be as physically active as their abilities and conditions allow. They can do exercises that maintain or improve balance if they are at risk of falling. Older adults should determine their level of effort for physical activity relative to their level of fitness and those with chronic conditions can understand whether and how their conditions affect their ability to do regular physical activity safely.

Regular physical activity is essential for healthy aging. Adults aged 65 years and older gain substantial health benefits from regular physical activity, and these benefits continue to occur throughout their lives. Promoting physical activity for older adults is especially important because this population is the least physically active of any age group.

Older adults are a varied group. Most, but not all, have one or more chronic conditions, and these conditions vary in type and severity. All have experienced a loss of physical fitness with age, some more than others. This diversity means that some older adults can run several miles, while others struggle to walk several blocks.

This section provides guidance about physical activity for adults aged 65 years and older. It focuses on physical activity beyond baseline activity. The Guidelines seek to help older adults select types and amounts of physical activity appropriate for their abilities. The Guidelines for older adults are also appropriate for adults younger than age 65 who have chronic conditions and those with a low level of fitness.

Meeting Guidelines

For adults aged 65 and older who are fit and have no limiting chronic conditions, the guidance in this section is essentially the same as that provided for adults. Like the Guidelines for other adults, those for older adults mainly focus on two types of activity: aerobic and muscle-strengthening. In addition, these Guidelines discuss the addition of *balance training* for older adults at risk of falls. Each type provides important health benefits.

Aerobic Activity

People doing aerobic activities move large muscles in a rhythmic manner for a sustained period. Brisk walking, jogging, biking, dancing, and swimming are all examples of aerobic activities. This type of activity is also called endurance activity. Aerobic activity makes a person's heart beat more rapidly to meet the demands of the body's movement.

Over time, regular aerobic activity makes the heart and cardiovascular system stronger and fitter.
When putting the Guidelines into action, it's important to consider the total amount of activity, as well as how often to be active, for how long, and at what intensity.

How much total activity a week?

Older adults should aim to do at least 2 hours and 30 minutes of moderate-intensity physical activity a week, or an equivalent amount (75 minutes or 1 hour and 15 minutes) of vigorous-intensity activity. Older adults can also do an equivalent amount of activity by combining moderate- and vigorous intensity activity. As is true for younger people, greater amounts of physical activity provide additional and more extensive health benefits to people aged 65 years and older.
No matter what its purpose—walking the dog, taking a dance or exercise class, or bicycling to the store—aerobic activity of all types counts toward the Guidelines.

How many days a week and for how long?

Aerobic physical activity should be spread throughout the week. Research studies consistently show that activity performed on at least 3 days a week produces health benefits. Spreading physical activity across at least 3 days a week may help to reduce the risk of injury and avoid excessive fatigue. Episodes of aerobic activity count toward meeting the Guidelines if they last at least 10 minutes and are performed at moderate or vigorous intensity.

These episodes can be divided throughout the day or week. For example, a person who takes a brisk 15-minute walk twice a day on every day of the week would easily meet the minimum Guideline for aerobic activity.

How intense?

Older adults can meet the Guidelines by doing relatively moderate-intensity activity, relatively vigorous intensity activity, or a combination of both. Time spent in light activity (such as light housework) and sedentary activities (such as watching TV) do not count. The relative intensity of aerobic activity is related to a person's level of cardio respiratory fitness.

•   Moderate-intensity activity requires a medium level of effort. On a scale of 0 to 10, where sitting is 0 and the greatest effort possible is 10, moderate-intensity activity is a 5 or 6 and produces noticeable increases in breathing rate and heart rate.

•   Vigorous-intensity activity is a 7 or 8 on this scale and produces large increases in a person's breathing and heart rate.

A general rule of thumb is that 2 minutes of moderate intensity activity count the same as 1 minute of vigorous-intensity activity. For example, 30 minutes of moderate-intensity activity a week is roughly same as 15 minutes of vigorous-intensity activity.

Muscle-Strengthening Activities

At least 2 days a week, older adults should do muscle strengthening activities that involve all the major muscle groups. These are the muscles of the legs, hips, chest, back, abdomen, shoulders, and arms. Muscle-strengthening activities make muscles do more work than they are accustomed to during activities of daily life. Examples of muscle-strengthening activities include lifting weights, working with resistance bands, doing calisthenics using body weight for resistance (such as push-ups, pull-ups, and sit-ups), climbing stairs, carrying heavy loads, and heavy gardening.

Muscle-strengthening activities count if they involve a moderate to high level of intensity, or effort, and work the major muscle groups of the body. Whatever the reason for doing it, any muscle-strengthening activity counts toward meeting the Guidelines. For example, muscle-strengthening activity done as part of a therapy or rehabilitation program can count.

No specific amount of time is recommended for muscle strengthening, but muscle-strengthening exercises should be performed to the point at which it would be difficult to do another repetition without help. When resistance training is used to enhance muscle strength, one set of 8 to 12 repetitions of each exercise is effective, although two or three sets may be more effective. Development of muscle strength and endurance is progressive over time. This means that gradual increases in the amount of weight or the days per week of exercise will result in stronger muscles.

Balance Activities for Older Adults at Risk of Falls

Older adults are at increased risk of falls if they have had falls in the recent past or have trouble walking. In older adults at increased risk of falls, strong evidence shows that regular physical activity is safe and reduces the risk of falls. Reduction in falls is seen for participants in programs that include balance and moderate-intensity muscle-strengthening activities for 90 minutes (1 hour and 30 minutes) a week plus moderate-intensity walking for about 1 hour a week.

Preferably, older adults at risk of falls should do balance training 3 or more days a week and do standardized exercises from a program demonstrated to reduce falls. Examples of these exercises include backward walking, sideways walking, heel walking, toe walking, and standing from a sitting position. The exercises can increase in difficulty by progressing from holding onto a stable support (like furniture) while doing the exercises to doing them without support. It's not known whether different combinations of type, amount, or frequency of activity can reduce falls to a greater degree. Tai chi exercises also may help prevent falls.

Meeting the Guidelines

Older adults have many ways to live an active lifestyle that meets the Guidelines. Many factors influence decisions to be active, such as personal goals, current physical activity habits, and health and safety considerations.

Healthy older adults generally do not need to consult a health-care provider before becoming physically active. However, health-care providers can help people attain and maintain regular physical activity by providing advice on appropriate types of activities and ways to progress at a safe and steady pace.

Adults with chronic conditions should talk with their health-care provider to determine whether their conditions limit their ability to do regular physical activity in any way. Such a conversation should also help people learn about appropriate types and amounts of physical activity.

Inactive Older Adults

Older adults should increase their amount of physical activity gradually. It can take months for those with a low level of fitness to gradually meet their activity goals. To reduce injury risk, inactive or insufficiently active adults should avoid vigorous aerobic activity at first. Rather, they should gradually increase the number of days a week and duration of moderate-intensity aerobic activity. Adults with a very low level of fitness can start out with episodes of activity less than 10 minutes and slowly increase the minutes of light-intensity aerobic activity, such as light-intensity walking.

Older adults who are inactive or who don't yet meet the Guidelines should aim for at least 2 and half hours a week of relatively moderate-intensity physical activity. Getting at least 30 minutes of relatively moderate intensity physical activity on 5 or more days each week is a reasonable way to meet these Guidelines. Doing muscle-strengthening activity on 2 or 3 non-consecutive days each week is also an acceptable and appropriate goal for many older adults.

Active Older Adults

Older adults who are already active and meet the Guidelines can gain additional and more extensive health benefits by moving beyond the 150-minute-a-week minimum to 300 or more minutes a week of relatively moderate-intensity aerobic activity. Muscle strengthening activities should also be done at least 2 days a week.

Older Adults With Chronic Conditions

Older adults who have chronic conditions that prevent them from doing the equivalent of 150 minutes of moderate-intensity aerobic activity a week should set physical activity goals that meet their abilities. They should talk with their health-care provider about setting physical activity goals. They should avoid an inactive lifestyle. Even 60 minutes (1 hour) a week of moderate-intensity aerobic activity provides some health benefits.

Special Considerations

Doing a Variety of Activities, Including Walking In working toward meeting the Guidelines, older adults are encouraged to do a variety of activities. This approach can make activity more enjoyable and may reduce the risk of overuse injury. Older adults also should strongly consider walking as one good way to get aerobic activity. Many studies show that walking has health benefits, and it has a low risk of injury. It can be done year-round and in many settings.

Physical Activity for Older Adults Who Have Functional Limitations

When a person has lost some ability to do a task of everyday life, such as climbing stairs, the person has a functional limitation. In older adults with existing functional limitations, scientific evidence indicates that regular physical activity is safe and helps improve functional ability.

Resuming Activity after an Illness or Injury

Older adults may have to take a break from regular physical activity because of illness or injury, such as the flu or a muscle strain. If these interruptions occur, older adults should resume activity at a lower level and gradually work back up to their former level of activity.

Flexibility, Warm-up, and Cool-down

Older adults should maintain the flexibility necessary for regular physical activity and activities of daily life. When done properly, stretching activities increase flexibility. Although these activities alone have no known health benefits and have not been demonstrated to reduce risk of activity-related injuries, they are an appropriate component of a physical activity program.

However, time spent doing flexibility activities by themselves does not count toward meeting aerobic or muscle-strengthening Guidelines.

Research studies of effective exercise programs typically include warm-up and cool-down activities. Warm-up and cool-down activities before and after physical activity can also be included as part of a personal program. A warm-up before moderate- or vigorous-intensity aerobic activity allows a gradual increase in heart rate and breathing at the start of the episode of activity. A cool-down after activity allows a gradual decrease at the end of the episode.

Time spent doing warm-up and cool-down may count toward meeting the aerobic activity Guidelines if the activity is at least moderate intensity (for example, walking briskly to warm-up for a jog). A warm-up for muscle-strengthening activity commonly involves doing exercises with less weight than during the strengthening activity.

Physical Activity in a Weight-Control Plan The amount of physical activity necessary to successfully maintain a healthy body weight depends on caloric intake and varies considerably among older adults. To achieve and maintain a healthy body weight, older adults should first do the equivalent of 2 and half hours of moderate-intensity aerobic activity each week. If necessary, older adults should increase their weekly minutes of aerobic physical activity gradually over time and decrease caloric intake to a point where they can achieve energy balance and a healthy weight.

Some older adults will need a higher level of physical activity than others to maintain a healthy body weight. Some may need more than the equivalent of 5 hours a week of moderate-intensity activity. It is possible to achieve this level of activity by gradually increasing activity over time.

Older adults who are capable of relatively vigorous intensity activity and need a high level of physical activity to maintain a healthy weight should consider some relatively vigorous-intensity activity as a means of weight control. This approach is more time-efficient than doing only moderate-intensity activity. However, high levels of activity are not feasible for many older adults. These adults should achieve a level of physical activity that is sustainable and safe. If further weight loss is needed, these older adults should achieve energy balance by regulating caloric intake.

It is important to remember that all activities "count" for energy balance. Active choices, such as taking the stairs rather than the elevator or adding short episodes of walking to the day, are examples of activities that can be helpful in weight control.

Key Guidelines for Older Adults

The following Guidelines are the same for adults and older adults:

•   All older adults should avoid inactivity. Some physical activity is better than none, and older adults who participate in any amount of physical activity gain some health benefits.

•   For substantial health benefits, older adults should do at least 150 minutes (2 hours and 30 minutes) a week of moderate-intensity, or 75 minutes (1 hour and 15 minutes) a week of vigorous-intensity aerobic physical activity, or an equivalent combination of moderate- and vigorous-intensity aerobic activity. Aerobic activity should be performed in episodes of at least 10 minutes, and preferably, it should be spread throughout the week.

•   For additional and more extensive health benefits, older adults should increase their aerobic physical activity to 300 minutes (5 hours) a week of moderate-intensity, or 150 minutes a week of vigorous-intensity aerobic physical activity, or an equivalent combination of moderate- and vigorous-intensity activity. Additional health benefits are gained by engaging in physical activity beyond this amount.

•   Older adults should also do muscle-strengthening activities that are moderate or high intensity and involve all major muscle groups on 2 or more days a week, as these activities provide additional health benefits.

The following Guidelines are just for older adults:

•   When older adults cannot do 150 minutes of moderate-intensity aerobic activity a week because of chronic conditions, they should be as physically active as their abilities and conditions allow.
•   Older adults should do exercises that maintain or improve balance if they are at risk of falling.

•   Older adults should determine their level of effort for physical activity relative to their level of fitness.

•   Older adults with chronic conditions should understand whether and how their conditions affect their ability to do regular physical activity safely.

Examples of Aerobic and Muscle Strengthening Physical Activities for Older Adults

The intensity of these activities can be either relatively moderate or relatively vigorous, depending on an older adult's level of fitness

Aerobic

- Walking
- Dancing
- Swimming
- Water aerobics
- Jogging
- Aerobic exercise classes
- Bicycle riding (stationary or on a path)
- Some activities of gardening, such as raking and pushing a lawn mower
- Tennis
- Golf (without a cart

Muscle-Strengthening

- Exercises using exercise bands, weight machines, hand-held weights

- Calisthenic exercises (body weight provides resistance to movement)
- Digging, lifting, and carrying as part of gardening
- Carrying groceries
- Some yoga exercises
- Some tai chi exercise

Examples

The following examples show how different people with different living circumstances and levels of fitness can meet the Guidelines for older adults.

- **Mary: A 75-Year-Old Woman Living Independently in Her Own Home**

Mary gets the equivalent of 180 minutes (3 hours) of moderate-intensity aerobic activity each week, plus muscle-strengthening activity 3 days a week.

- She participates regularly in an exercise class at her local senior center. The class meets Mondays, Wednesdays, and Fridays. It includes 30 minutes of aerobic dance, which she can do at moderate intensity, as well as 20 minutes of strength training, a 5-minute warm-up, a 5-minute cool-down, and some stretching exercises.

- On most Sundays, she visits her favorite park and walks a loop trail with several friends, which takes them about 45 minutes. The trail is hilly, so about 30 minutes of the walk is moderate-intensity walking for her, and about 15 minutes is vigorous intensity (the 15 minutes of vigorous intensity counts as 30 minutes of moderate-intensity walking).

- She adds at least an additional 30 minutes of walking each week in different ways. For example, she walks her grandson to school, she walks to her friends' homes, or she walks at the mall during shopping trips.

- **Manuel: An 85-Year-Old Man Living in an Assisted-Living Facility**

Manuel, who has problems with falls, gets about 70 minutes (1 hour and 10 minutes) of aerobic activity each week and has an individualized strength-training program. He cannot do 2 and half hours of moderate intensity physical activity because of his chronic conditions, but he is being as physically active as his condition allows.

- To reduce the risk of falls, a physical therapist has prescribed an individualized exercise program. This program includes 3 days a week (30 minutes each session) of strength- and balance-training exercises. Manuel uses ankle weights for lower body muscle strengthening exercises and does a series of balance exercises. He does this program with the assistance
of a residential aide.

- Manuel's residence includes a garden with walking paths and benches. He has gradually increased his physical activity to walking about 10 minutes each day. On some days he can walk more than on others, but he tries to walk a little every day. The plan is for him to sustain this level of activity for several weeks.

- After he builds strength and his balance improves, Manuel will consider increasing his level of activity and joining an exercise class specially designed to reduce the risk of falls in older people.

- **Anthony: A 65-Year-Old Man Living in a Retirement Community**

Anthony has been active and it all his life. He does over 2 and half hours of relatively vigorous-intensity activity each week, plus muscle-strengthening activities on 3 days.

- Six days a week, Anthony gets up early and runs 3 miles, which takes about 30 minutes.

- With help from staff at his community's fitness facility, Anthony designed a weight-lifting program using weight machines. He does this program on 3 day

Guidelines for Woman during Pregnancy and the Postpartum Period

 Healthy women who are not already highly active or doing vigorous-intensity activity should get at least a little over 2 hours of moderate-intensity aerobic activity a week during pregnancy and the postpartum period. Preferably, this activity should be spread throughout the week. Also, pregnant women who habitually engage in vigorous-intensity aerobic activity or who are highly active can continue physical activity during pregnancy and the postpartum period, provided that they remain healthy and discuss with their health-care provider how and when activity should be adjusted over time.

Although physical activity has many health benefits, injuries and other adverse events do sometimes happen. The most common injuries affect the musculoskeletal system (the bones, joints, muscles, ligaments, and tendons). Other adverse events can also occur during activity, such as overheating and dehydration. On rare occasions, people have heart attacks during activity.

The good news is that scientific evidence strongly shows that physical activity is safe for almost everyone. Moreover, the health benefits of physical activity far outweigh the risks.

Still, people may hesitate to become physically active because of concern they'll get hurt. For these people, there is even more good news: They can take steps that are proven to reduce their risk of injury and adverse events.

The Guidelines in this section provide advice to help people do physical activity safely. Most advice applies to people of all ages. Specific guidance for particular age groups and people with certain conditions is also provided.

Physical Activity Is Safe for Almost Everyone

Most people are not likely to be injured when doing moderate-intensity activities in amounts that meet the Physical Activity Guidelines. However, injuries and other adverse events do sometimes happen. The most common problems are musculoskeletal injuries. Even so, studies show that only one such injury occurs for every 1,000 hours of walking for exercise, and fewer than four injuries occur for every 1,000 hours of running.

Both physical fitness and total amount of physical activity affect risk of musculoskeletal injuries. People who are physically it have a lower risk of injury than people who are not. People who do more activity generally have a higher risk of injury than people who do less activity. So what should people do if they want to be active and safe? The best strategies are to:

- Be regularly physically active to increase physical fitness; and

- Follow the other guidance in this chapter (especially increasing physical activity gradually over time) to minimize the injury risk from doing medium to high amounts of activity.

Following these strategies may reduce overall injury risk. Active people are more likely to have an activity related injury than inactive people. But they appear less likely to have non-activity-related injuries, such as work-related injuries or injuries that occur around the home or from motor vehicle crashes.

Choose Appropriate Types and Amounts of Activity

People can reduce their risk of injury by choosing appropriate types of activity. As the table shows, the safest activities are moderate intensity and low impact, and don't involve purposeful collision or contact.

Walking for exercise, gardening or yard work, bicycling or exercise cycling, dancing, swimming, and golf are activities with the lowest injury rates. In the amounts commonly done by adults, walking (a moderate intensity and low-impact activity) has a third or less of the injury risk of running (a vigorous-intensity and higher impact activity).

The risk of injury for a type of physical activity can also differ according to the purpose of the activity. For example, recreational bicycling or bicycling for transportation leads to fewer injuries than training for and competing in bicycle races.

People who have had a past injury are at risk of injuring that body part again. The risk of injury can be reduced by performing appropriate amounts of activity and setting appropriate personal goals. Performing a variety of different physical activities may also reduce the risk of overuse injury.

Increase Physical Activity Gradually Over Time

Scientific studies indicate that the risk of injury to bones, muscles, and joints is directly related to the gap between a person's usual level of activity and a new level of activity. The size of this gap is called the amount of overload. Creating a small overload and waiting for the body to adapt and recover reduces the risk of injury. When amounts of physical activity need to be increased to meet the Guidelines or personal goals, physical activity should be increased gradually over time, no matter what the person's current level of physical activity.

The following recommendations give general guidance for inactive people and those with low levels of physical activity on how to increase physical activity:

•   Use relative intensity (intensity of the activity relative to a person's fitness) to guide the level of effort for aerobic activity.

•   Generally start with relatively moderate-intensity aerobic activity. Avoid relatively vigorous-intensity activity, such as shoveling snow or running. Adults with a low level of fitness may need to start with light activity, or a mix of light- to moderate intensity activity.

•   First, increase the number of minutes per session (duration), and the number of days per week (frequency) of moderate-intensity activity. Later, if desired, increase the intensity.

•   Pay attention to the relative size of the increase in physical activity each week, as this is related to injury risk. For example, a 20-minute increase each week is safer for a person who does 200 minutes a week of walking (a 10 percent increase), than for a person who does 40 minutes a week (a 50 percent increase).

The available scientific evidence suggests that adding a small and comfortable amount of light- to moderate intensity activity, such as 5 to15 minutes of walking per session, 2 to 3 times a week, to one's usual activities has a low risk of musculoskeletal injury and no known risk of severe cardiac events. Because this range is rather wide, people should consider three factors in individualizing their rate of increase: age, level of fitness, and prior experience.

Age

The amount of time required to adapt to a new level of activity probably depends on age. Youth and young adults probably can safely increase activity by small amounts every week or 2. Older adults appear to require more time to adapt to a new level of activity, in the range of 2 to 4 weeks.

Level of Fitness

Less it adults are at higher risk of injury when doing a given amount of activity, compared to fitter adults. Slower rates of increase over time may reduce injury risk. This guidance applies to overweight and obese adults, as they are commonly less physically it.

Prior Experience

People can use their experience to learn to increase physical activity over time in ways that minimize the risk of overuse injury. Generally, if an overuse injury occurred in the past with a certain rate of progression, a person should increase activity more slowly the next time.

Take Appropriate Precautions

Taking appropriate precautions means using the right gear and equipment, choosing safe environments in which to be active, following rules and policies, and making sensible choices about how, when, and where to be active.
Use Protective Gear and Appropriate Equipment

Using personal protective gear can reduce the frequency of injury. Personal protective gear is something worn by a person to protect a specific body part. Examples include helmets, eyewear and goggles, shin guards, elbow and knee pads, and mouth guards.

Using appropriate sports equipment can also reduce risk of injury. Sports equipment refers to sport or activity-specific tools, such as balls, bats, sticks, and shoes. For the most benefit, protective equipment and gear should be:

- The right equipment for the activity;

- Appropriately fitted

- Appropriately maintained; and

- Used consistently and correctly.

Be Active in Safe Environments

People can reduce their injury risks by paying attention to the places they choose to be active. To help themselves stay safe, people can look for:

- Physical separation from motor vehicles, such as sidewalks, walking paths, or bike lanes;

- Neighborhoods with traffic-calming measures that slow down traffic;

- Places to be active that are well-lighted, where other people are present, and that are well-maintained (no litter, broken windows);

- Shock-absorbing surfaces on playgrounds;

- Well-maintained playing fields and courts without holes or obstacles;

- Breakaway bases at baseball and softball fields; and

- Padded and anchored goals and goal posts at soccer and football fields.

Follow Rules and Policies That Promote Safety

Rules, policies, legislation, and laws are potentially the most effective and wide-reaching way to reduce activity-related injuries. To get the benefit, individuals should look for and follow these rules, policies, and laws. For example, policies that promote the use of bicycle helmets reduce the risk of head injury among cyclists. Rules against diving into shallow water at swimming pools prevent head and neck injuries.

Make Sensible Choices About How, When, and Where To Be Active

A person's choices can obviously influence the risk of adverse events. By making sensible choices, injuries and adverse events can be prevented. Consider weather conditions, such as extremes of heat and cold. For example, during very hot and humid weather, people lessen the chances of dehydration and heat stress by:

- Exercising in the cool of early morning as opposed to mid-day heat;

- Switching to indoor activities (playing basketball in the gym rather than on the playground);

- Changing the type of activity (swimming rather than playing soccer)

- Lowering the intensity of activity (walking rather than running); and

- Paying close attention to rest, shade, drinking enough fluids, and other ways to minimize effects of heat.

Exposure to air pollution is associated with several adverse health outcomes, including asthma attacks and abnormal heart rhythms. People who can modify the location or time of exercise may wish to reduce these risks by exercising away from heavy traffic and industrial sites, especially during rush hour or times when pollution is known to be high. However, current evidence indicates that the benefits of being active, even in polluted air, outweigh the risk of being inactive.

Advice from Health-Care Providers

The protective value of a medical consultation for persons with or without chronic diseases who are interested in increasing their physical activity level is not established. People without diagnosed chronic conditions (such as diabetes, heart disease, or osteoarthritis) and who do not have symptoms (such as chest pain or pressure, dizziness, or joint pain) do not need to consult a health-care provider about physical activity.

Inactive people who gradually progress over time to relatively moderate-intensity activity have no known risk of sudden cardiac events, and very low risk of bone, muscle, or joint injuries. A person who is habitually active with moderate-intensity activity can gradually increase to vigorous intensity without needing to consult a health-care provider. People who develop new symptoms when increasing their levels of activity should consult a health-care provider.

Health-care providers can provide useful personalized advice on how to reduce risk of injuries. For people who wish to seek the advice of a health-care provider, it is particularly appropriate to do so when contemplating vigorous-intensity activity, because the risks of this activity are higher than the risks of moderate-intensity activity.

The choice of appropriate types and amounts of physical activity can be affected by chronic conditions. People with symptoms or known chronic conditions should be under the regular care of a health-care provider. In consultation with their provider, they can develop a physical activity plan that is appropriate for them. People with chronic conditions typically find that moderate-intensity activity is safe and beneficial. However, they may need to take special precautions. For example, people with diabetes need to pay special attention to blood sugar control and proper footwear during activity.

Women who are pregnant and those who've recently had a baby should be under the regular care of a health-care provider. Moderate-intensity physical activity is generally safe for women with uncomplicated pregnancies, but women should talk with their provider about how to adjust the amounts and types of activity while they are pregnant and right after the baby's birth.

During pregnancy, women should avoid:

•   Doing activities that involve lying on their back after the first trimester of pregnancy;
and

•   Doing activities with high risk of falling or abdominal trauma, including contact or collision sports, such as horseback riding, soccer, basketball, and downhill skiing.

Examples on gradually Increasing Physical Activity over Time:

Here are two examples that show how people at different ages, levels of fitness, and levels of experience can safely become more active over time.

Bill: A Man Who Has Been Inactive for Many Years

Bill wants to work his way up to the equivalent of 3 hours to 3 hours and 30 minutes of walking a week. On weekdays he has time for up to 45 minutes of walking, and he plans to do something physically active each weekend. He decides to start with walking because it is moderate intensity and has a low risk of injury.

•   The first week, Bill starts at a low level. He walks 10 minutes a day 3 days a week. Sometimes he divides the 10 minutes a day into two sessions. He prefers to alternate rest days and active days. (Total = 30 minutes a week.)

•   Between weeks 3 and 8, Bill increases duration by adding 5 minutes a day and continues walking on 3 non-consecutive days each week. The weekly increase is 15 minutes. (Week 3 total = 45 minutes. Week 8 total = 120 minutes or 2 hours.)

•   In week 9, Bill adds another day of moderate intensity activity on the weekend, and starts doing a variety of activities, including biking, hiking, and an aerobics class. Gradually increasing the minutes of activity, by week 12 he is doing 60 minutes or more of moderate-intensity activity on the weekend.

Reaching his goal: Over 3 months, Bill has increased to a total of 180 moderate-intensity minutes a week.

Kim: An Active Woman

Kim currently does 150 minutes (2 hours and 30 minutes) a week of moderate-intensity activity.
She wants to work up to at least the equivalent of 300 minutes (5 hours) of moderate-intensity
activity a week. She also wants to shift some of that moderate intensity activity to vigorous-intensity activity. Her current 150 minutes a week includes:

•   Thirty minutes of mowing the grass 1 day a week;

•   Thirty minutes of brisk walking 4 days a week; and

•   Fifteen minutes of muscle-strengthening exercises 2 days a week.

Increasing frequency and duration:

- Over a month, Kim adds walking on another weekday, and she gradually adds 15 minutes of moderate-intensity activity on each of the 5 walking days each week. This provides an additional 105 minutes (1 hour and 45 minutes) of moderate intensity activity.

Increasing intensity:

- Over the next month, Kim decides to replace some walking with jogging. Instead of walking 45 minutes, she walks for 30 minutes and jogs for 15 minutes on each weekday, providing the equivalent of 300 minutes a week of moderate-intensity physical activity from her walking and jogging.

Reaching her goal: After these increases, Kim is doing a total of 180 minutes of moderate-intensity activity each week (walking and mowing) and also doing 75 minutes (1 hour and 15 minutes) of vigorous intensity jogging. One minute of vigorous-intensity activity is about the same as 2 minutes of moderate intensity activity, so she is now doing the equivalent of 330 moderate-intensity minutes (5 hours and 30 minutes) a week. She has more than met her goal.

Additional Physical Activity for Women During Pregnancy and the Postpartum Period

Physical activity during pregnancy benefits a woman's overall health. For example, moderate-intensity physical activity by healthy women during pregnancy maintains or increases cardio respiratory fitness.

Strong scientific evidence shows that the risks of moderate-intensity activity done by healthy women during pregnancy are very low, and do not increase risk of low birth weight, preterm delivery, or early pregnancy loss. Some evidence suggests that physical activity reduces the risk of pregnancy complications, such as preeclampsia and gestational diabetes, and reduces the length of labor, but this evidence is not conclusive.

During a normal postpartum period, regular physical activity continues to benefit a woman's overall health. Studies show that moderate-intensity physical activity during the period following the birth of a child increases a woman's cardio respiratory fitness and improves her mood. Such activity does not appear to have adverse effects on breast milk volume, breast milk composition, or infant growth.

Physical activity also helps women achieve and maintain a healthy weight during the postpartum period, and when combined with caloric restriction, helps promote weight loss.

Explaining the Guidelines

Women who are pregnant should be under the care of a health-care provider with whom they can discuss how to adjust amounts of physical activity during pregnancy and the postpartum period. Unless a woman has medical reasons to avoid physical activity during pregnancy, she can begin or continue moderate-intensity aerobic physical activity during her pregnancy and after the baby is born.

When beginning physical activity during pregnancy, women should increase the amount gradually over time. The effects of vigorous-intensity aerobic activity during pregnancy have not been studied carefully, so there is no basis for recommending that women should begin vigorous-intensity activity during pregnancy.

Women who habitually do vigorous-intensity activity or high amounts of activity or strength training should continue to be physically active during pregnancy and after giving birth. They generally do not need to drastically reduce their activity levels, provided that they remain healthy and discuss with their health-care provider how to adjust activity levels during this time.

During pregnancy, women should avoid doing exercises involving lying on their back after the first trimester of pregnancy. They should also avoid doing activities that increase the risk of falling or abdominal trauma, including contact or collision sports, such as horseback riding, downhill skiing, soccer, and basketball.

Key Guidelines for Women during Pregnancy and the Postpartum Period

•   Healthy women who are not already highly active or doing vigorous-intensity activity should get at least 150 minutes (2 hours and 30 minutes) of moderate-intensity aerobic activity per week during pregnancy and the postpartum period. Preferably, this activity should be spread throughout the week.

•   Pregnant women who habitually engage in vigorous-intensity aerobic activity or are highly active can continue physical activity during pregnancy and the postpartum period, provided that they remain healthy and discuss with their health-care provider how and when activity should be adjusted over time.

Guidelines for Adults with Disabilities

Adults with disabilities, who are able to, can get at least 2 hours a week of moderate-intensity, or 75 minutes a week of vigorous-intensity aerobic activity, or an equivalent combination of moderate-and vigorous-intensity aerobic activity. Aerobic activity should be performed in episodes of at least 10 minutes, and preferably, it should be spread throughout the week.

Adults with disabilities, who are able to, can also do muscle-strengthening activities of moderate or high intensity that involve all major muscle groups on 2 or more days a week, as these activities provide additional health benefits. When adults with disabilities are not able to meet the Guidelines, they should engage in regular physical activity according to their abilities and should avoid inactivity. Adults with disabilities should consult their healthcare provider about the amounts and types of physical activity that are appropriate for their abilities

Physical Activity for People with Disabilities

The benefits of physical activity for people with disabilities have been studied in diverse groups. These groups include stroke victims, people with spinal cord injury, multiple sclerosis, Parkinson's disease, muscular dystrophy, cerebral palsy, traumatic brain injury, limb amputations, mental illness, intellectual disability, and dementia.

Overall, the evidence shows that regular physical activity provides important health benefits for people with disabilities. The benefits include improved cardiovascular and muscle fitness, improved mental health, and better ability to do tasks of daily life. Sufficient evidence now exists to recommend that adults with disabilities should get regular physical activity.

In consultation with their health-care providers, people with disabilities should understand how their disabilities affect their ability to do physical activity. Some may be capable of doing medium to high amounts of physical activity, and they should essentially follow the Guidelines for adults.

Some people with disabilities are not able to follow the Guidelines for adults. These people should adapt their physical activity program to match their abilities, in consultation with their health-care providers. Studies show that physical activity can be done safely when the program is matched to an individual's abilities.

Meeting the Guidelines

People with disabilities are encouraged to get advice from professionals with experience in physical activity and disability because matching activity to abilities can require modifying physical activity in many different ways. Some people with disabilities also need help with their exercise program. For example, some people may need supervision when performing muscle strengthening activities, such as lifting weights.

Key Guidelines for Adults With Disabilities

•   Adults with disabilities, who are able to, should get at least 150 minutes per week (2 hours and 30 minutes) of moderate-intensity, or 75 minutes (1 hour and 15 minutes) per week of vigorous-intensity aerobic activity, or an equivalent combination of moderate- and vigorous-intensity aerobic activity. Aerobic activity should be performed in episodes of at least 10 minutes, and preferably, it should be spread throughout the week.

•   Adults with disabilities, who are able to, should also do muscle-strengthening activities of moderate or high intensity that involve all major muscle groups on 2 or more days per week, as these activities provide additional health benefits.

•   When adults with disabilities are not able to meet the above Guidelines, they should engage in regular physical activity according to their abilities and should avoid inactivity.

•   Adults with disabilities should consult their health-care providers about the amounts and types of physical activity that are appropriate for their abilities.

Guidelines for People with Chronic Medical Conditions

Adults with chronic conditions obtain important health benefits from regular physical activity.

When adults with chronic conditions do activity according to their abilities, physical activity is safe. Adults with chronic conditions should be under the care of a health-care provider. People with chronic conditions and symptoms should consult their health-care provider about the types and amounts of activity appropriate for them.

Adults with chronic conditions should engage in regular physical activity because it can help promote their quality of life and reduce the risk of developing new conditions. The type and amount of physical activity should be determined by a person's abilities and the severity of the chronic condition. Three examples are provided below to illustrate the benefits of physical activity for persons with chronic conditions.

For many chronic conditions, physical activity provides therapeutic benefits and is part of recommended treatment for the condition. However, this chapter does not discuss therapeutic exercise or rehabilitation.

Example 1. Physical Activity for Adults With Osteoarthritis

Osteoarthritis is a common condition in older adults, and people can live many years with osteoarthritis. People with osteoarthritis are commonly concerned that physical activity can make their condition worse. Osteoarthritis can be painful and cause fatigue, making it hard to begin or
maintain regular physical activity. Yet people with this condition should get regular physical activity to lower their risk of getting other chronic diseases, such as heart disease or type 2 diabetes, and to help maintain a healthy body weight.

Strong scientific evidence indicates that both aerobic activity and muscle-strengthening activity provide therapeutic benefits for persons with osteoarthritis. When done safely, physical activity does not make the disease or the pain worse. Studies show that adults with osteoarthritis can expect improvements in pain, physical function, quality of life, and mental health with regular physical activity.

People with osteoarthritis should match the type and amount of physical activity to their abilities and the severity of their condition. Most people can usually do moderate-intensity activity for 150 minutes (2 hours and 30 minutes) a week or more, and may choose to be active 3 to 5 days a week for 30 to 60 minutes per episode. Some people with arthritis can safely do more than 150 minutes of moderate-intensity activity each week and may be able to tolerate equivalent amounts of vigorous-intensity activity. Health-care providers typically counsel people with osteoarthritis to do activities that are low impact, not painful, and have low risk of joint injury. Swimming, walking, and strength training are good examples of this type of activity.

Example 2. Physical Activity for Adults With Type 2 Diabetes

Physical activity in adults with type 2 diabetes shows how important it can be for people with a chronic disease to be active. Physical activity has important therapeutic effects in people with diabetes, but it is also routinely recommended to reduce risk of other diseases and help promote a healthy body weight.

For example, strong scientific evidence shows that physical activity protects against heart disease in people with diabetes. Moderate-intensity activity for about 2 and half hours a week helps to substantially lower the risk of heart disease. A person who moves toward 5 hours or more of moderate-intensity activity a week gets even greater benefit.

Adults with chronic conditions should work with their health-care providers to adapt physical activity so that it is appropriate for their condition. For example, people with diabetes must be careful to monitor their blood glucose and avoid injury to their feet.

Example 3. Physical Activity for Cancer Survivors

With modern treatments, many people with cancer can either be cured or survive for many years, living long enough to be at risk of other chronic conditions, such as high blood pressure or type 2 diabetes. Some cancer survivors are at risk of recurrence of the original cancer. Some have experienced side effects of the cancer treatment.

Like other adults, cancer survivors should engage in regular physical activity for its preventive benefits. Physical activity in cancer survivors can reduce risk of new chronic diseases. Further, studies suggest physically active adults with breast or colon cancer are less like to die prematurely or have a recurrence of the cancer. Physical activity may also play a role in reducing adverse effects of cancer treatment.

Cancer survivors, like other adults with chronic conditions, should consult their health-care providers to match their physical activity plan to their abilities and health status.

Key Messages for People with Chronic Medical Conditions

• Adults with chronic conditions obtain important health benefits from regular physical activity.

• When adults with chronic conditions do activity according to their abilities, physical activity is safe.

• Adults with chronic conditions should be under the care of health-care providers. People with chronic conditions and symptoms should consult their health-care providers about the types and amounts of activity appropriate for them.

Additional Guidelines for Safe Physical and Healthy Lifestyle

Lift your spirits with this simple back bending yoga sequence

If you thought "heartache" and "heavy-hearted" were just evocative turns of phrase, think again. In fact, research shows that sudden emotional stress can release hormones that prevent the heart from pumping normally. Even watching a sad movie can reduce arterial blood flow. And if emotions affect the body so acutely, then it seems logical that the body could in turn influence our emotions.

"The heart is a vulnerable space," says Kimberly Wilson, author of *Hip, Tranquil Chick: A Guide to Life On and Off the Yoga Mat*. "Backbends help expand the heart center and help you exude confidence and grace." In other words, backbends ease breathing, improve posture, and reduce stress by releasing tension held in the tissues of the whole chest and lung region of the body. So the next time you need to kick the bad-day blues, try this sequence of heart-opening backbends from Wilson's book.

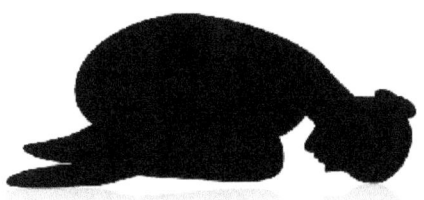

Child's Pose:

Relieves stress and fatigue as it stretches the lower back and hips

1. Sit on your heels with your big toes touching and hands resting on your thighs.

2. Lower your belly and chest to rest between your knees, bringing your forehead to the floor.

3. Relax your arms back beside your shins, palms facing up.

4. Soften your breath by taking 5 to 10 long, deep inhalations and exhalations.

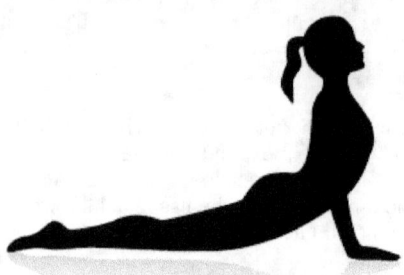

Cobra Pose, Modified:

Boosts energy and mood as it strengthens the back of the body

1. Slowly slide forward from Child's Pose to lie face down.

2. Press your toes and forehead gently into the floor. Rest your palms lightly on the floor on either side of your chest with fingertips pointing forward and elbows bent and hugging in toward your ribcage.

3. Inhale and lift your chest from the heart, pressing only very lightly into your palms and mostly using your back strength to hold your shoulders and chest up.

4. Soften your shoulders. Then lift your hands off the floor completely, broadening across your collarbones and reaching your heart up. Take a couple of deep, slow breaths here.

5. Then as you exhale, place your palms back down and gently lower your chest to floor

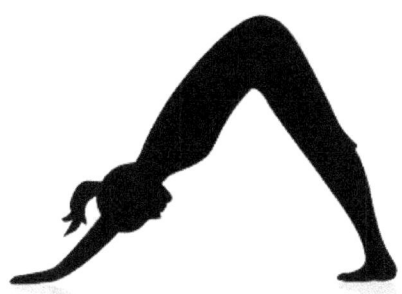

Downward-Facing Dog Pose

Reduces fatigue and focuses the mind as it strengthens and stretches most of the body

1. From Cobra, come onto all fours. Separate your knees to hip-width apart, move your wrists slightly forward of your shoulders, and curl your toes under.

2. Exhale and spread your fingers wide, press evenly through your palms, and lift your knees to reach your hips toward the ceiling. Keep your legs slightly bent.

3. Push the tops of your thighs back so your body looks like an inverted "V" Slowly start to straighten your legs as much as feels appropriate for you, without locking your knees.

4. Gently move your chest back toward your thighs until your ears are even with your upper arms. And keep lifting your hips away from your heels and wrists.

Hint: Your heels don't necessarily ever need to touch the floor in this pose. But if you're aiming for that, reach your heels away from your head first and then down to elongate rather than yank your leg muscles.

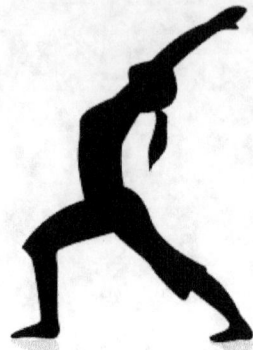

Warrior I Pose

Eases stress and anxiety as it strengthens the legs and core

1. From Downward-Facing Dog, pivot your left heel down to the floor so your toes are pointing out to the left.

2. Step your right foot forward between your hands, lining your front heel up with your back.

3. Inhale and lift your arms overhead, shoulder-width apart, palms facing each other.

4. Exhale as you bend your front knee to 90 degrees and turn your hips toward your right leg.

5. Inhale as you reach your arms up higher and maybe back slightly for a gentle bend in the upper back. Hold for 3 to 10 slow, deep breaths.

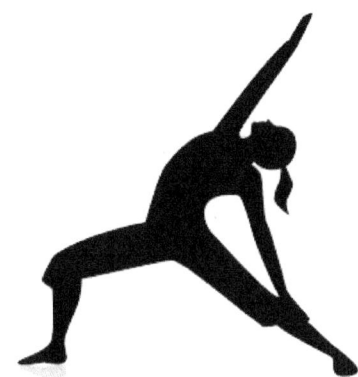

Reverse Warrior Pose

Energizes the body and focuses a scattered mind while stretching and strengthening the legs and abs

1. From Warrior I, turn your hips to face the side, keeping your right knee bent deeply.

2. Lower your left hand to rest gently on your left leg and turn your right palm toward the ceiling as you reach your right arm up overhead, reaching back behind you without moving your legs. Let your left hand slide down toward your left ankle.

3. Look up at the ceiling if it doesn't bother your neck. Stay here for 3 to 5 deep breaths.

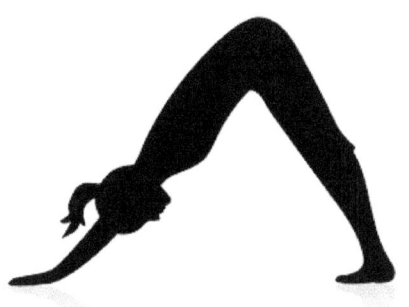

Transition

From Reverse Warrior, return to Downward-Facing Dog Pose and transition to the other side

1. Repeat steps 4 and 5 with your left leg forward this time.

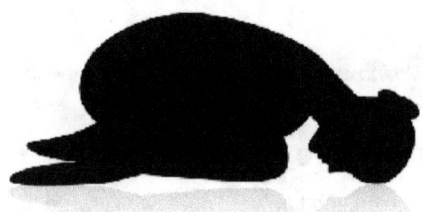

Child's Pose

Take a break! You've earned it

1. From Downward-Facing Dog, drop your knees to the floor and rest your hips on your heels.

2. Let your arms relax, palms facing up, next to your legs.

3. Take 10 deep breaths, feeling each inhalation fill the back of your body with breath.

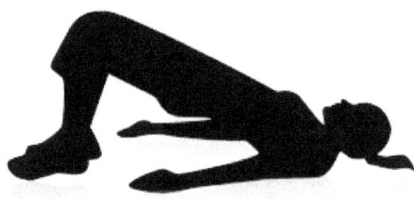

Bridge Pose
Boosts mood and mitigates anxiety while increasing the flexibility of the spine

1. From Child's Pose, roll up to a seated position and drop your hips over to the left to sit on the floor.

2. Extend your legs straight out in front of you and slowly roll down onto your back.

3. Bend your knees and place your feet flat on the floor close to your butt, palms facing down.

4. Inhale as you lift your hips. Interlace your hands beneath you and press your shoulders and upper arms into the floor.

5. Lift your hips higher and point your tailbone toward your knees, pressing firmly into your feet. Squeeze your thighs toward each other. Hold for 5 to 7 breaths before slowly lowering back to the floor

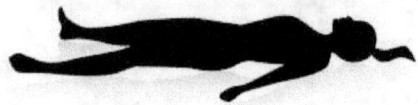

Supported Corpse Pose
Relaxes tension and rejuvenates both the body and mind

1. Place a folded blanket, bolster, or firm pillow either lengthwise behind you or across your mat so that when you lie back it hits you under the tip of your shoulder blades, your mid-back.

2. Then lie back, letting your body sink into and open around the support. End in a supported pose on your back with a folded blanket under the length of the spine to help arch the upper and middle back, and lengthen the lower back.

3. Move your arms a comfortable distance away from your body and anything else around you. Turn your palms to face up.

4. Separate your legs a natural distance apart. Relax your feet and let them roll open.

5. Finally, do a mental scan from head to toe: Where are you holding tension? Release it from every part of your body—including your heart and head.

10 Model-Worthy Yoga Poses

Try this series of poses, all with a specific benefit, created by cover model Claudia Rocafort
By Amanda Junker
While we can't fit enough sun salutations in a day to make our bodies start to compete with our Venezuelan cover model's, these 10 yoga poses will still leave you feeling strong, flexible, and maybe even photogenic. Claudia Rocafort has practiced Kundalini, Ashtanga, and Hatha yoga for about 10 years, ever since she stopped dancing at age

22. "Yoga helps me strengthen and regain the flexibility I lost when I stopped dancing," she says.

Rocafort has taught yoga at a holistic spa in Venezuela and says she makes sure to do at least 6 or 7 basic asana postures every day. She used those basic postures, plus a few extra yoga poses, to develop her Cover Model Workout--an at home yoga routine you can practice to help make you look and feel cover model-worthy. "Each pose has a benefit," she says of the sequence. "The sun salutations are wonderful because they incorporate the flow and focused movement that I find integral. The rest of the sequence gives me focus and balance and allows me to really let go."

1. Cat and Cow poses

With your hands and knees on the floor, breathe in, arch the back tucking your stomach in, tucking your tailbone in, sucking your belly button in toward the spine and your neck loose, head hanging down in Cat pose. Exhale, dropping the belly, arching the back so your tailbone lifts up, your head is up and your shoulders are open, chest forward in Cow pose. Repeat, alternating between Cat and Cow between 10 or 15 times. This really warms up the spine, releases the hamstring and gets you into a nice rhythm for your practice.

2. Sun Salutation Series

Stand up into Mountain Pose, both feet planted on the ground, shoulder-width apart, spine straight, standing tall. Inhale, stretching your arms up parallel overhead. As you exhale, fold down into a forward bend, folding at the waist and releasing the entire upper body so you hang loose stretching the back and hamstrings. Then inhale, arch your back up into a half lift, hinging your torso up so it's at a right angle to your legs and you are looking forward. Then exhale, releasing back down into the forward bend and holding for one or two breaths. On an inhale, straighten your body back up, extending your arms out and up as you stand so the fingertips meet, touching overhead. Look upward, extending the neck and back to elongate the spine, then release your hands down into mountain pose so you are again standing grounded in mountain pose. Repeat this cycle five times.

3. Triangle

Stand with your legs 4 feet apart. Raise your arms shoulder-height, parallel to the floor with your palms down. Turn your left foot in about 45 degrees, and your right foot about 90 degrees. Your front heel should bisect the back foot. Bending from your hips, extend your torso to the right directly over your right leg, placing your right arm on a block behind your right foot. Stretch your left arm toward the ceiling, keeping your shoulders stacked in a straight line. Hold four or five breaths then straighten your torso and transition to Side Angle Lunge.

4. Side Angle Lunge

Bend your right leg about 90 degrees, so your right knee is directly over your right heel and your right foot is pointed straight ahead. Your left leg should be stretched straight back, with your foot turned in about 45 degrees and planted firmly on the mat. Cross your right arm over the front leg, extended straight down with your palm facing out. Beginners can keep the left arm on the left side, or for more of a challenge, straighten the left arm up to the ceiling or over your ear, all the way forward.

5. Side Angle Bind

For a more intense torso-twisting, leg-strengthening yoga pose, you can transition into Side Angle Bind. Reach your right arm back through your legs and drop your left arm back behind your body clasp your right hand. Hold for three or four breaths, or as long as feels comfortable, elongating the spine and keeping your back straight. When you release from side angle repeat steps 3 through 5 on the left side.

6. Pigeon

Begin in Downward Facing Dog. Bring right leg forward to the ground, placing right knee behind right wrist, and allowing right heel to draw in toward groin--the closer it is to the groin, the gentler the stretch. Using the arms to support body weight, chest and lengthen spine as you stay here for as long as you comfortably can. Return to Down Dog and repeat on opposite side.

7. Camel

Kneeling, with your body erect and your knees directly beneath your hips, and toes curling under. Stack your hips on top of your knees, your shoulders atop your hips, and your ears atop your shoulders. Then place the palms of your hands on the small of your back, fingertips facing up. If that is uncomfortable, the fingertips can face the floor. As you inhale, inflate the chest and feel your breastbone rise, floating the ribcage up and off the waist. Then continue to lift the upper back up and over an imaginary ball behind you until you begin to reach one hand and then the other toward the heels. You should arrive in your deepest arch only in the upper back when both hands rest comfortably on your heels or props. Take five full, complete breaths, letting the head drop back; if that strains the neck, tuck the chin and relax the face muscles.

8. Crow

From a deep squat, place your hands flat on the floor in front of you so they are shoulder width apart. Come to your tiptoes and walk your feet closer to your body. Then slowly bring your weight forward onto the hands and off the feet until your knees touch your upper arms. As you deepen the bend in your elbows, inch the knees up above the elbows, bringing them as close to the armpits as possible. Transfer the weight fully onto the arms, squeeze your elbows in, tighten your abs, and press your shins into your forearms, causing your feet to float up behind you. You might want to rest in Child's Pose for a few breaths after Crow.

9. Shoulderstand

Lie on your back with arms by your side. Bend your knees and rock your legs up, bringing your knees to your forehead and placing your hands under your hips to support them, keeping your elbows on the floor. Slowly straighten your legs into the air, balancing for 8 to 10 breaths, then slowly release your knees and roll gently back onto the floor.

10. Savasana

Lie on your back, completely relaxed, with your arms resting on your sides or palms on your belly. Rest in this pose for at least a 10 minute meditation

Stay Young with Tai Chi

How can something this easy be such potent medicine? Discover the power of this ancient exercise
By Caroline Bollinger is *Prevention's* fitness editor.

(Sept. 5, 2006) -- Georgina Duggan just knew she'd wind up with arthritis in her spine. "My mother and one of my brothers had back pain from arthritis, so when it started to bother me, I figured it was something I'd have to live with," says the 60-year-old retiree in Mississauga, Ontario. But unlike her family, she isn't suffering anymore. Thanks to an unusual kind of remedy, she's off all her painkillers and feels better than she has in years.

Initially, Duggan went to a chiropractor several times a week for relief. "It helped some, but I got tired of having to go so often." Her physician suggested the ancient art of tai chi. Says Duggan: "He thought the combination of slow movements, meditation, and breathing would help strengthen my spine and increase my flexibility. I thought, Why not?"

After all, the Chinese have been maintaining their health with tai chi for centuries. And today, more than 200,000 Americans take tai chi classes in health clubs--a number that has doubled in the past 4 years, says Rosemary Lavery, a spokesperson for the International Health, Racquet, and Sports club Association.

Part of tai chi's appeal is that it doesn't really feel like exercise. "It offers cardiovascular benefits similar to brisk walking or low-impact aerobics, but it's much easier on the body," says Ruth Taylor-Piliae, Phd, RN, a tai chi researcher and postdoctoral fellow at Stanford University School of Medicine. "It's good for people who might not be capable of strenuous activity." The stances require you to shift your weight slowly from one foot to the other--and you have to maintain control throughout the moves. "This keeps your mind focused, improves balance, and strengthens your body," Taylor-Piliae says.

Indeed, tai chi offers stellar health benefits. For instance, a recent review of 47 studies published in the Archives of Internal Medicine suggested that tai chi can lower blood pressure; increase flexibility, strength, and balance; and decrease stress, anxiety, and depression. Find out what tai chi might do for you from people who are already practicing.

"My blood pressure dropped."
--Linda Bowers, 57, former administrative assistant, Kansas City, MO

When layoffs left Linda Bowers without health insurance 3 years ago, she made the difficult decision to go off her blood pressure medication. Instead, Bowers got serious about daily tai chi to maintain a healthier blood pressure. At her annual checkup--which she paid for out-of-pocket--she was pleasantly surprised to see her BP remain at a steady 134/82.

Low-intensity exercise can work wonders on blood pressure. Researchers at the Stanford Prevention Research Center recently had 39 sedentary seniors do 60 minutes of tai chi three times a week for 12 weeks. On average, the group lowered their resting systolic blood pressure (the larger number) by 13% to a healthier reading of 131 mm/Hg and decreased their resting diastolic BP by 10% to 77 mm/Hg--results similar to those from medication.

Granted, any aerobic exercise would have helped, "but studies indicate that the mental component of tai chi may offer an edge," says Taylor-Piliae, the lead researcher on the study. "Our theory is that the level of focus that tai chi requires triggers a relaxation response. That, in turn, helps reduce the volume of blood going to the heart, making the heart more efficient and thus lowering blood pressure."

"My stress plummeted."
--Sue Gurland, 62, acupuncturist, Boca Raton, FL

"When I get stressed, all the tension goes to my head and neck," says Sue Gurland. "Tai chi relieves my tension. I feel clearheaded and in a much lighter mood." Gurland, who has been practicing for 30 years, says the discipline has changed her outlook on life, too. Research suggests that her results are common.

Studies show the complex series of movements in tai chi reduce the body's level of cortisol, a stress hormone. In another Stanford study of 39 seniors, those who practiced an hour of tai chi 3 days a week for 12 weeks boosted their overall sense of well-being. By the end of the study, participants reported improvement in mood of about 12%--and a 13% decrease in stress.

"I don't get sick as much."
--Diane Rapaport, 67, writer and publisher, Burns, OR

"I used to have bronchitis three or four times a year," remembers Diane Rapaport. "It was awful." Since she started tai chi 6 years ago, however, she hasn't had so much as a sniffle. Experts believe tai chi decreases the release of catecholamine, a neurotransmitter that has been shown to dampen the immune system. A 2003 UCLA study found that a three-times-a-week routine enhanced T cell function by 45% after 4 months. (T cells attack virus-infected cells.)

Though the research looked specifically at the virus that causes shingles, "we believe tai chi would improve resistance to other viruses as well," says Michael Irwin, MD, lead author of the study and a professor of psychiatry at the Cousins Center for Psychoneuroimmunology at UCLA.

"Tai chi improved my balance."
--Bob Erler, 68, retired librarian, Bronx, NY

Six years ago, Bob Erler was diagnosed with Charcot-Marie-Tooth disease, a rare condition that reduces sensation in limbs, fingers, and toes--and caused Erler to frequently fall. Practicing tai chi about five times a week, however, has given him remarkable results: "I used to fall about twice a month. Last year, I fell just twice altogether," Erler says. "I've always liked to walk and keep active, but I became fearful after my diagnosis. Today, I'm confident and more trusting of my body."

Says Rhayun Song, PhD, an assistant professor of nursing at Daewon Science College in South Korea: "To prevent falls, you need balance and muscle strength, especially in the lower body." Tai chi seems to improve both. In Song's recent study of 59 seniors, the researcher found that those who did 35 minutes of tai chi three times a week for 12 weeks were only half as likely to fall as those who didn't practice the discipline.

Get started

Take a class - Many YMCAs, hospitals, and community centers offer them. Check out the Institute of Integral Qigong and Tai Chi to find an instructor in your area. (Qigong can vary from tai chi to the more vigorous kung fu.)

Start Your Fat-Burning Solutions from Experts
Five frustrated women beat a plateau and slim down for good

By Ann Hettinger, Ann Hettinger a freelance health writer and adjunct professor of magazine journalism at Syracuse University.

The facts are simple: To look fit and firm at any age, you have to strength-train, says Wayne Westcott, PhD, senior fitness research director at the South Shore YMCA in Quincy, MA. Women lose about 1/2 pound of muscle a year, beginning as early as in their 20s. But that's not inevitable. According to two studies Westcott conducted over 15 years of more than 2,800 women and men, on average, you can gain 3 pounds of muscle, lose 2 inches around your waist, and drop 4 pounds of fat- -without dieting --in 10 weeks by strength-training at least twice a week. Plus, new muscle revs metabolism. "A 3-pound muscle gain increases metabolism by about 7%, which translates to burning roughly 100 more calories a day," explains Westcott. The more muscle you have, the more calories you burn.

Here, Westcott (coauthor of *Get Stronger, Feel Younger*) and his associate Rita LaRosa Loud use his findings to help five women reshape their current toning routines with more impressive findings--up to 4 inches off their waists and 5 pounds down on the scale in just 8 weeks.

1. "I lift weights but my arms jiggle!" -Arnesse Brown

Arnesse regularly worked out 4 days a week, alternating between traditional 60-minute aerobic classes and 90-minute combo ones that included cardio, weights, and ad exercise. She also did a series of upper-body moves with 6- or 8-pound dumbbells. "I'm in my 40s and in good shape but not satisfied with my triceps," she says. "For someone who works out as much as I do, I'd like to see a little more definition."

Expert Rx: Change things up

Regular activity keeps you fit and healthy, but if you always do the same exercise with the same weight for the same number of reps, your muscles get bored. "Muscles adapt to repetitive movements and eventually stop developing," says Westcott. To help Arnesse bust her plateau, he suggested challenging her muscles with the following strategies:

Mix single- and multimuscle moves

To tone a specific area, your workout should include exercises that isolate a trouble spot (single-muscle moves) and those that also work the surrounding muscles. You'll get better results, says Westcott, because you're still training the target area but not overloading it to the point of injury.

Practice the 6-second rep

Lift for 2 counts, lower in 4--that's the breakdown that challenges you the most, says Westcott. The reason: Your muscles are strongest during the eccentric contraction, or lowering phase. "Slowing down this part of the exercise makes your muscles work significantly harder," he says.

Sample Workout
One set of 10 reps, 2 or 3 times per week

What you need: bench and set of dumbbells

Overhead Press

Firms shoulders, arms

Stand with feet hip width apart, abs tight, heels pressed into floor with dumbbells just above shoulders, palms facing forward and elbows out to sides (shown right). Lift dumbbells straight up in 2 counts, keeping elbows slightly bent, then slowly lower to start position in 4 counts.

Chest Press

Firms chest, shoulders, triceps

Lie face up on bench, feet on floor, holding dumbbells with arms extended above chest and palms forward. Bend elbows out to sides as you lower weights toward chest in 4 counts (don't let elbows drop below bench). Press weights up to start position in 2 counts.

Bent Over Row

Firms upper back, biceps
Kneel with right knee and right hand on bench, left foot on floor, and abs tight with back straight from top of head to butt. Hold dumbbell in left hand with arm extended under shoulder, palm facing bench. Pull elbow toward ceiling in 2 counts as you lift weight to rib cage, then lower to start position in 4 counts.

Standing Triceps Extension

Firms triceps
Stand with feet hip width apart, abs tight, heels pressed into floor, and arms extended above head holding dumbbell with palms facing each other. Lower dumbbells straight behind head in 4 counts, keeping elbows close to ears; lift up to start position in 2 counts.

Arnesse's results

"I was excited to lose almost 5 pounds in 6 weeks, but the best part is there's a noticeable change in my upper body. When I'm wearing a T shirt, I can see the difference in the backs of my arms. The muscles aren't bulky at all, they just look nice."

2."I walk but I'm still flabby" -Mary Godley, 39
Although Mary logged 30 to 45 minutes of brisk walking two or three times a week, she still couldn't get rid of her post baby flab more than a year after the birth of her daughter. "I used to wear formfitting shirts without feeling self-conscious," she says. "Now, I always choose loose clothing and cringe if I have to put on anything without sleeves."

Expert Rx: Add strength-training

Cardio exercise, such as walking and jogging, are great for burning fat and keeping your heart and lungs healthy, explains Westcott, but they do little to build the muscle that gives you a toned look. For that, you need to lift weights. How to get started:

Use heavy-enough weights

The amount you lift should be light enough for you to complete at least 8 reps of an exercise using good form, but heavy enough that by the 12th rep, your muscles are so fatigued you can't imagine doing another one.

Trade dumbbells for a weighted ball

Mary had tried lifting weights in the past but gave it up because it was "time-consuming and boring." To spark her interest, Westcott created a routine using a weighted medicine ball (sporting goods stores; $25 to $35). "It's less intimidating than dumbbells, and many people find that it feels more like play than exercise," he says. Holding the ball with both hands is also simpler than trying to synchronize dumbbell movements with each hand.

Sample Workout
One set of 8 to 12 reps, 3 times per week

What you need: weighted ball

Knee Lift with Pull Down

Firms shoulders, arms, oblique, butt, thighs

Stand tall with feet staggered, left leg about 1 foot in front of right, abs in, and holding medicine ball with both hands over left shoulder . Slowly pull ball diagonally across body toward right hip, twisting right, while lifting right knee toward left shoulder. Return to start and repeat. Do all reps on left leg, then switch sides and repeat.

Step Hop

Firms abs, butt, legs

Stand tall, feet hip-width apart, abs in, and knees slightly bent. Hold medicine ball in front of belly, elbows close to sides. Keeping ball steady, hop to right, balancing on right leg while lifting left knee up to touch ball. Pause 1 count, then hop onto left foot, balancing as you lift right knee up to ball. Pause 1 count. (That's 1 rep.)

Arm and Leg Swing

Firms shoulders, obliques, butt, inner and outer thighs

Stand tall, feet hip-width apart, abs in, and knees slightly bent. Hold medicine ball in front of belly, elbows close to sides. In a slow, controlled motion, lift left leg across right while bringing medicine ball toward left side of body; keep torso facing forward. Pause 1 count, squeezing inner thigh. Then slowly swing left leg out to left side while bringing ball to right side of body. Pause 1 count, contracting outer thigh and gluts. (That's 1 rep.) Do all reps on right leg, then switch sides and repeat. Tip: Try not to use momentum or arch lower back.

Crunch Roll

Firms abs

Lie face up, knees bent, and feet flat on floor. Hold medicine ball on belly. Exhale as you lift head, neck and shoulders off floor, rolling ball up thighs toward knees. Pause at top for 1 count; inhale and roll ball back down thighs to return to start. Mary's results "The moves were new to me, so I didn't get bored, and in just 3 weeks, I noticed my pants felt looser. After 8 weeks, I lost 4 inches off my waist and dropped almost 5 pounds."

3."I don't see results with strength training classes" -Tara Healy, 45
When she began losing muscle tone about 5 years ago, Tara started taking an hour-long sculpting class at her gym three times a week using hand weights and doing lots of reps. But after a year and a half, she saw minimal, and then eventually no more, improvement.

Expert Rx: Focus on quality, not quantity

Doing numerous reps with lighter weights doesn't have the same muscle-building effect as doing fewer reps with a heavy weight, says Westcott. Tara can do the same moves from class, but following these tips:

Practice proper form

When you churn through dozens of reps, you may start to get tired and sloppy. Instead, focus on every stage of the exercise -no bouncing, slumping, or jerking allowed.

Lift more

To keep muscles challenged, gradually increase both the reps and weight over several weeks. Choose a weight you can lift for 12 reps with proper form. Then move up to a heavier weight next time (say, from 5 to 7 pounds). Start with 8 reps at the new weight, and slowly work back up to 12 reps; then bump up the weight again.

Tara's results

"After 6 weeks, I lost 3 inches around my waist. I developed bad habits in class, but the form fixes were worth the effort because I feel and look more toned. My new routine takes less time, and I get better results."

4. "Crunches and yoga aren't flattening my belly" -Sheila Nutt, 59
Ever since she hit her mid-40s, Sheila has watched the pounds gradually pile around her middle--even with her committed routine of 100 crunches and yoga stretches, three mornings a week.

Expert Rx: Target all ab muscles

Crunches are great to shape the abs, but you also have to work the hip flexors and obliques to really tone your midsection. How to tweak the crunch, plus some new toning tricks:

Slow down

"When you speed through any exercise, your body's momentum propels the movement, so the muscles don't have to work as hard and you don't get results," says Westcott. Each crunch should take a full 7 seconds--3 seconds to lift, a 1-second hold at the top, and 3 seconds to lower.

Do strength-building yoga moves

Poses that require you to support your entire body weight, like the boat or plank, may be among the best at strengthening your core because you have to engage your deep_abdominal muscles, often for 30 to 60 seconds.

Sample Workout
Two sets; 4 reps, work up to 16 (except half boat and plank), every other day

What you need: cushioned surface

Knee-Up Crunch

Firms abs and hip flexors Lie face up, legs extended, heels on floor, and hands behind head. Lift shoulders, point right elbow forward, and raise right knee to meet elbow; keep left leg on floor. Repeat on other side. (That's 1 rep.)

Half Boat

Firms abs

Sit on floor, knees bent, and feet down. Lean back, engaging abs, and lift feet, keeping back straight and knees bent with shins parallel to floor. Reach forward with hands, keeping arms at should level. Balance for 30 counts.

Push Pull

Firms abs and obliques

Lie face up, hands behind head, and legs extended 45 degrees off floor. Lift shoulders and twist upper body to right, bringing right knee toward left elbow; then left knee to right elbow. (That's 1 rep.) Plank Firms abs, lower back Lie face down, resting on forearms, hands flat. Push off floor; keep weight on arms and toes. Keep back in a straight line from head to heels. Hold for 30 counts.

Sheila's results

"Once I started slowing down my crunches and adding the other ab moves to my routine, I felt the muscles all around my midsection working. Within 3 weeks, I could button my favorite pants again. After 6 weeks, my waistline shrank 1 1/2 inches."

5. "I'm too busy to work out!" -Kelly Fleming, 44
With three children under age 11, Kelly found it hard to maintain a regular routine. "I'd plan to go to the gym on a Saturday morning but end up having to drive one of the kids someplace instead," she says. When she did work out, she'd often overdo it to make up for missed sessions and then wouldn't feel like going back for weeks.

Expert Rx: do shorter, regular at-home workouts

To keep fit, Kelly needs consistency, not the occasional all-or-nothing routine. "Her marathon exercise sessions may actually have interfered with her progress," says Westcott. You need time to recover after weight training, which causes microscopic tears in muscle tissue that your body then rebuilds. "One extra-long workout can deplete your energy for days, energy your body needs to get stronger," Westcott says. To create a routine to fit any busy schedule, he suggests these time-saving tips:

Stick to 20-minute strength-training sessions

"According to our studies, it's just enough time to work every body part and make a difference, but not so much that it feels like a burden," says Westcott.

Make basic moves harder

You don't need equipment to challenge your muscles--simple variations or a shift in body position can either work the target muscle harder or bring more muscles in play. (See the next page for some ideas to "make it harder.")

Do these exercises as a circuit, 10 reps per move, going from one exercise to the next without taking a rest; complete the circuit 3 times through. Do this circuit 2 or 3 times per week.

What you need: seat, cushioned surface

Step-Up
Firms butt, legs

Stand facing sturdy seat, feet together, and arms at sides. Place right foot up on seat, knee bent 90 degrees. Pushing into right heel, step left foot onto seat next to right. Slowly step left foot down, then right. Repeat, placing left foot on seat and stepping up with right. (That's 1 rep.)

Make it harder: Add a high knee lift at the top of your step.

Knee-Up Crunch

Firms abs and hip flexors

Lie face up, legs extended, heels on floor, and hand behind head. Lift shoulders, point right elbow forward, and raise right knee to meet elbow; keep left leg on floor. Repeat on other side. (That's 1 rep.)

Push-Up
Firms chest, arms, abs

Begin in a modified push-up position, hands on floor under shoulders and knees down, forming a straight line from head to hips. Lower chest toward floor, bending elbows 90 degrees; hold for 1 count and press up to start.

Make it harder: Do a full push-up with straight legs.

Squat
Firms thighs, butt

Stand with feet hip-width apart, and arms at sides. Bend knees 90 degrees as if sitting in a chair behind you; keep weight over heels (lift arms forward to help you counterbalance). Hold for 1 count and squeeze glutes as you stand back to start position. Make it harder: Jump up between each rep, landing in squat position.

Dips
Firms triceps

Sit on edge of seat and grip front edge with hands shoulder-width apart. Extend legs straight in front of body with heels on floor. Lift hips forward, keeping body close to seat. Exhaling, slowly bend elbows 90 degrees behind you, lowering hips toward floor. Inhaling, push back up and repeat; don't lock elbows at the top.

Make it harder: Lift one leg for first 5 reps; switch legs for second 5 reps.

Kelly's Results

"Working out doesn't seem like a chore anymore. I saved so much time, and I felt firmer in just 2 weeks. I was even more thrilled to lose 2 1/2 pounds and 1/2 inch off my waist after 6 weeks."

12 Ways to Lower Blood Pressure Naturally

Reducing high blood pressure without drugs is easier than you think.

High blood pressure is one of the most preventable conditions.

But it plays a contributing role in more than 15% of deaths in the United States, according to a new Harvard study. Although it causes no symptoms, HBP boosts the risks of leading killers such as heart attack and stroke, as well as aneurysms, cognitive decline, and kidney failure. In fact, 28% of Americans have high blood pressure and don't know it, according to the American Heart Association. If you haven't had yours checked in 2 years, see a doctor.

Fortunately, most people can reduce their blood pressure without medication. First get to a healthy weight. Then add these strategies.

1. Go for power walks
Hypertensive patients who walked at a brisk pace lowered pressure by almost 8 mmhg over 6 mmhg. Exercise helps the heart use oxygen more efficiently, so it doesn't work as hard to pump blood. Get a vigorous cardio workout of at least 30 minutes on most days of the week. Try increasing speed or distance so you keep challenging your ticker.

2. Breathe deeply
Slow breathing and meditative practices such as qigong, yoga, and tai chi decrease stress hormones, which elevate renin, a kidney enzyme that raises blood pressure. Try 5 minutes in the morning and at night. Inhale deeply and expand your belly. Exhale and release all of your tension.

3. Pick potassium-rich produce
Loading up on potassium-rich fruits and vegetables is an important part of any blood pressure–lowering program, says Linda Van Horn, PhD, RD, professor of preventive medicine at Northwestern University Feinberg School of Medical. Aim for potassium levels of 2,000 to 4,000 mg a day, she says. Top sources of potassium-rich produce include sweet potatoes, tomatoes, orange juice, potatoes, bananas, kidney beans, peas, cantaloupe, honeydew melon, and dried fruits such as prunes and raisins.

4. Read food labels for sodium

Certain groups of people—the elderly, African Americans, and those with a family history of high blood pressure—are more likely than others to have blood pressure that's particularly salt (or sodium) sensitive. But because there's no way to tell whether any one individual is sodium sensitive, everyone should lower his sodium intake, says Eva Obarzanek, PhD, a research nutritionist at the National Heart, Lung, and Blood Institute. How far? To 1,500 mg daily, about half the average American intake, she says. (Half a teaspoon of salt contains about 1,200 mg of sodium.)

Cutting sodium means more than going easy on the saltshaker, which contributes just 15% of the sodium in the typical American diet. Watch for sodium in processed foods, Obarzanek warns. That's where most of the sodium in your diet comes from, she says. Season foods with spices, herbs, lemon, and salt-free seasoning blends.

5. Indulge in dark chocolate

Dark varieties contain flavanols that make blood vessels more elastic. In one study, 18% of patients who ate it every day saw blood pressure decrease. Have 1/2 ounce daily (make sure it contains at least 70% cocoa).

6. Take a supplement

In a review of 12 studies, researchers found that coenzyme Q10 reduced blood pressure by up to 17 mmhg over 10 mmhg. The antioxidant, required for energy production, dilates blood vessels. Ask your doctor about taking a 60 to 100 mg supplement up to 3 times a day

7. Drink alcohol—but not too much

According to a review of 15 studies, the less you drink, the lower your blood pressure will drop—to a point. A study of women at Boston's Brigham and Women's Hospital, for example, found that light drinking (defined as one-quarter to one-half a drink per day for a woman) may actually reduce blood pressure more than no drinks per day. One "drink" is 12 ounces of beer, 5 ounces of wine, or 1.5 ounces of spirits.

Other studies have also found that moderate drinking—up to one drink a day for a woman, two for a man—can lower risks of heart disease. "High levels of alcohol are clearly detrimental," says Obarzanek. "But moderate alcohol is protective of the heart. If you are going to drink, drink moderately."

8. Go decaf
Scientists have long debated the effects of caffeine on blood pressure. Some studies have shown no effect, but one from Duke University Medical Center found that caffeine consumption of 500 mg—roughly three 8-ounce cups of coffee—increased blood pressure by 4 mmhg, and that effect lasted until bedtime. For reference, 8 ounces of drip coffee contain 100 to 125 mg; the same amount of tea, 50 mg; an equal quantity of cola, about 40 mg.

Caffeine can raise blood pressure by tightening blood vessels and by magnifying the effects of stress, says Jim Lane, PhD, associate research professor at Duke and the lead author of the study. "When you're under stress, your heart starts pumping a lot more blood, boosting blood pressure," he says. "And caffeine exaggerates that effect." If you drink a lot of joe, pour more decaf to protect your ticker.

9. Take up tea
Lowering high blood pressure is as easy as one, two, tea: Study participants who sipped 3 cups of a hibiscus tea daily lowered systolic blood pressure by 7 points in 6 weeks on average, say researchers from Tufts University—results on par with many prescription medications. Those who received a placebo drink improved their reading by only 1 point.

The phytochemicals in hibiscus are probably responsible for the large reduction in high blood pressure, say the study authors. Many herbal teas contain hibiscus; look for blends that list it near the top of the chart of ingredients—this often indicates a higher concentration per serving

10. Work (a little) less
Putting in more than 41 hours per week at the office raises your risk of hypertension by 15%, according to a University of California, Irvine, study of 24,205 California residents. Overtime makes it hard to exercise and eat healthy, says Haiou Yang, PhD, the lead researcher. It may be difficult to clock out super early in today's tough economic times, but try to leave at a decent hour—so you can go to the gym or cook a healthy meal—as often as possible. Set an end-of-day message on your computer as a reminder to turn it off and go home.

11. Relax with music

Need to bring down your blood pressure a bit more than medication or lifestyle changes can do alone? The right tunes can help, according to researchers at the University of Florence in Italy. They asked 28 adults who were already taking hypertension pills to listen to soothing classical, Celtic, or Indian music for 30 minutes daily while breathing slowly. After a week, the listeners had lowered their average systolic reading by 3.2 points; a month later, readings were down 4.4 points.

12. Seek help for snoring

It's time to heed your partner's complaints and get that snoring checked out. Loud, incessant snores are one of the main symptoms of obstructive sleep apnea (OSA). University of Alabama researchers found that many sleep apnea sufferers also had high levels of aldosterone, a hormone that can boost blood pressure. In fact, it's estimated that half of all people with sleep apnea have high blood pressure.

If you have sleep apnea, you may experience many brief yet potentially life-threatening interruptions in your breathing while you sleep. In addition to loud snoring, excessive daytime tiredness and early morning headaches are also good clues. If you have high blood pressure, ask your doctor if OSA could be behind it; treating sleep apnea may lower aldosterone levels and improve BP.

Conclusion

To do physical activity safely and reduce the risk of injuries and other adverse events, people should understand the risks and yet be confident that physical activity is safe for almost everyone. People should choose to do types of physical activity that are appropriate for their current fitness level and health goals, because some activities are safer than others. They should increase physical activity gradually over time whenever more activity is necessary to meet guidelines or health goals. Inactive people should "start low and go slow" by gradually increasing how often and how long activities are done. They should protect themselves by using appropriate gear and sports equipment, looking for safe environments, following rules and policies, and making sensible choices about when, where, and how to be active.

If they however have chronic conditions or symptoms, they should be under the care of a health-care provider. People with chronic conditions and symptoms should consult their health-care provider about the types and amounts of activity appropriate for them.

Although this book focuses on the health benefits of physical activity, these benefits are not the only reason why people are active. Physical activities gives people a chance to have fun, be with friends and family, enjoy the outdoors, improve their personal appearance, and improve their fitness so that they can participate in more intensive physical activity or sporting events. Some people are active because they feel it gives them certain health benefits (such as feeling more energetic) that aren't yet conclusively proven for the general population.

The Guidelines encourage people to be physically active for any and all reasons that are meaningful for them. Nothing in the Guidelines is intended to mean that health benefits are the only reason to do physical activity.

The Guidelines focus on preventive effects of physical activity, which include lowering the risk of developing chronic diseases such as heart disease and type 2 diabetes. Physical activity also has beneficial therapeutic effects and is commonly recommended as part of the treatment for medical conditions.

To make these choices, adults need to set personal goals for physical activity. Setting these goals involves questions like, "How physically fit do I want to be?" "How important is it to me to reduce my risk of heart disease and diabetes?" "How important is it to me to reduce my risk of falls and hip fracture?" "How much weight do I want to lose and keep off?" People can meet the Guidelines and their own personal goals through different amounts and types of activity. Written materials, health-care providers, and fitness professionals can provide useful information and help people set and carry out specific goals.

References:

Centers for Disease Control and Prevention (CDC)
http://www.cdc.gov/ncipc/duip/preventadultfalls.htm

National Institutes of Health
http://nihseniorhealth.gov/exercise/toc.html

Office of the Surgeon General
http://www.surgeongeneral.gov/obesityprevention/index.html

President's Council on Physical Fitness and Sports
http://www.presidentschallenge.org

Division of Adolescent and School Health, CDC
http://www.cdc.gov/HealthyYouth/physicalactivity

Division of Nutrition, Physical Activity, and Obesity
(DNPAO), CDC
http://www.cdc.gov/nccdphp/dnpa/physical/index.htm

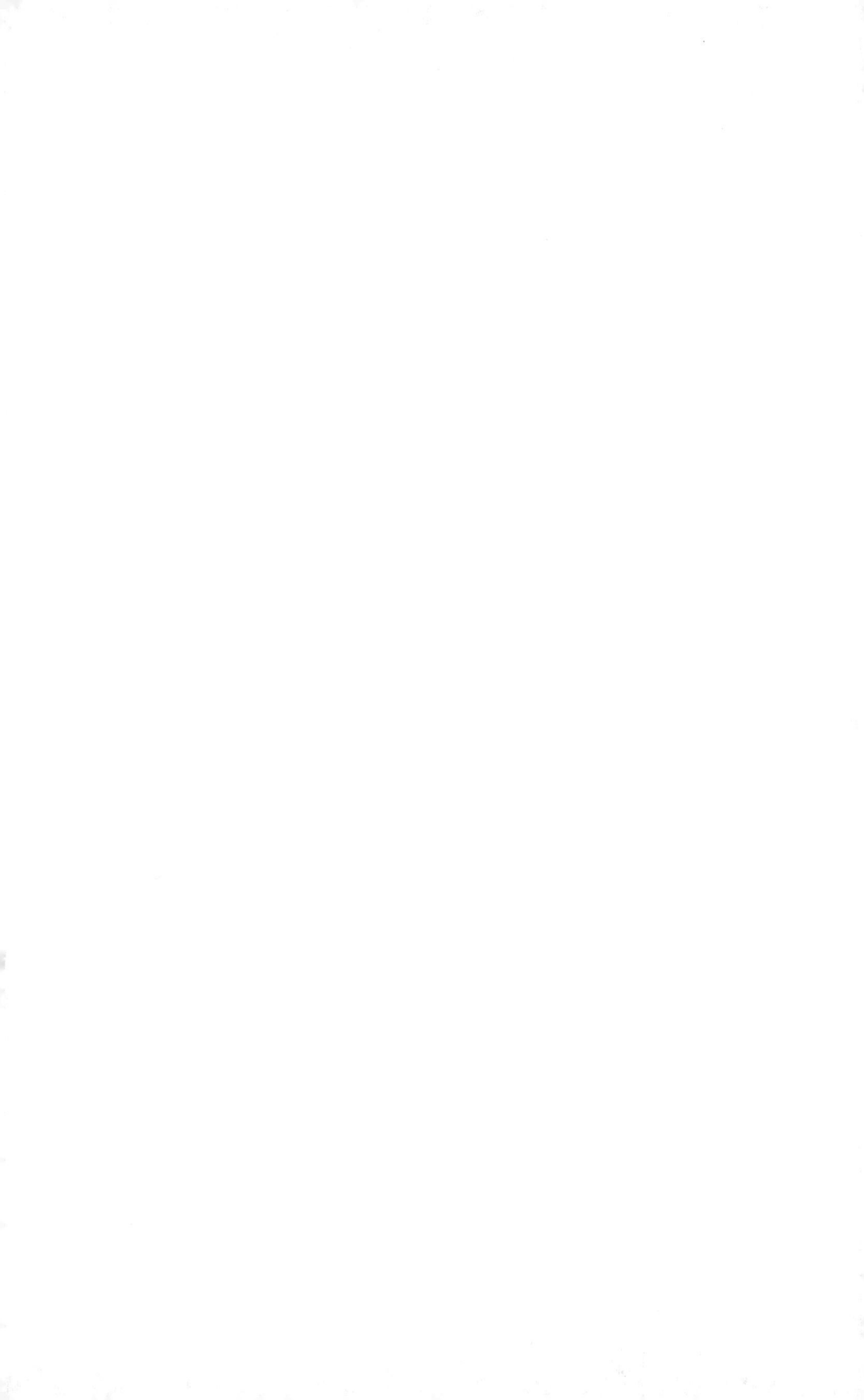